The Miracle
of
Maddie

Mariah Stubblefield

Cover image by Jessica Hollis Photography

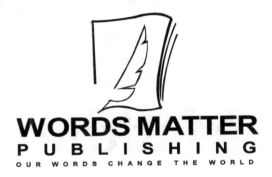

WORDS MATTER
PUBLISHING
OUR WORDS CHANGE THE WORLD

© 2020 by Mariah Stubblefield. All rights reserved.

Words Matter Publishing
P.O. Box 531
Salem, Il 62881
www.wordsmatterpublishing.com

ISBN: 978-1-949809-97-8

Library of Congress Catalog Card Number: 2020946550

Statistics about Maddie

—1,353— The number of days from when we started trying to have a baby until we held Maddie in our arms

—1,039— The number of days the lion sleeper hung in our bedroom before Maddie wore it.

— 270— The number of days Maddie lived in a freezer in Evansville as an embryo

— 45— The number of eggs retrieved from me throughout this process.

— 12— The day of the month Maddie's egg was retrieved (4/12/17), implanted in me (1/12/18) and her birthday (9/12/18)

—11— The number of eggs that made it to the embryo stage and were implanted in me.

—5— The number of times I have been pregnant

— 2— The number of ectopic pregnancies I had.

—1— The number of babies we hold in our arms—the number of embryos it took to make Maddie—Little is much when God is in it.

This book is called the Miracle of Maddie but truthfully our stories and faith start long before Maddie or our journey to get her....

Contents

MARIAH

I was born the year Kevin graduated from high school...don't think about that too much though or it will start to seem weird. My childhood was what I would consider the "normal American dream" so to speak. I was raised with two great parents, excelled in school and never needed for anything or wanted for much.

My childhood ended on April 20, 2005...I remember most details about that day like it was yesterday. When I got home from school that day the phone was ringing, I didn't quite make it in time to answer it, but it wasn't long before it rang again. My 19-year-old brother died that day. He was at my grandparents' house on his lunch break from work when he collapsed in the bathroom. His cause of death remains "unknown." I remember when I got to the ER that afternoon and my mom met me right outside the doors, I remember her telling me my brother was dead and I started screaming "NO, NO, NO...over and over again— my mom hugged me and leaned into my ear and said "You have to stop screaming" and at that moment I stopped screaming and grew up I also learned lessons that would prove extremely pertinent in our fight for Maddie 10 years later. That night I learned that life is not always fair, I learned that life keeps going even after extreme heartache I learned that you can learn to live again after tragedy. That's the thing about tragedy...life moves on.

I graduated from Belmont University in 2012 as an Occupational Therapist and started working at a hospital...where I met Kevin. It is still up for debate who asked who out and who was interested first, but ultimately Kevin and I went on our first date to Sonic in February of 2013. Kevin and I had been dating for a while when we began talking about the future. Marriage, life, kids...I remember the very date night that Kevin and I discussed having kids. To be honest the fact that Kevin was in a wheelchair had never really mattered to me until now. I worried that with Kevin's age and paralysis as factors we may never have kids and that was unacceptable to me. The night I told Kevin this I thought I was just talking to Kevin, but looking back now I wonder if I was talking to myself or the universe or maybe the Devil. I remember the conversation when I told Kevin that having a child was "a non-negotiable" factor for me. Throughout the course of the conversation, we discussed that we didn't have to have enough kids to create our own football team and we knew there were multiple ways to start a family, but that having A CHILD was non-negotiable. Kevin agreed. As you will learn throughout these chapters I am an excellent worrier and that is what I continued to do just that. As my relationship with Kevin grew continued to worry that we would have trouble having a child and that's when God told me to stop worrying. "Therefore do not be anxious about tomorrow, for tomorrow will be anxious for itself. Each day has enough trouble of its own." —Matthew 6:34 I didn't hear the audible voice of God, but stronger in my heart than I've ever felt or known anything I felt God telling me I would have A child. I would have chosen to have more children... I always thought at least 3 children, but I felt like God was preparing me to have one child and to quit worrying about it.

In that same Sonic parking lot from 1 year ago on February 22, 2014, Kevin asked me to marry him.

Facebook post-February 22, 2014

"I said YES!!!"

KEVIN

As much as I would say my childhood was ideal Kevin's would probably be the opposite. Kevin's parents got divorced when he was 12; however, he would probably say he wishes it would have happened sooner. His dad was not a nice man even on his best days (although sometimes Kevin will tell me a fond memory of his dad—though they are few and far between). I'm sure Kevin would describe his childhood as good even though he didn't have all the things others had.

Kevin was raised in church; however, in his high school years was quite the partier and his friends take great pleasure in telling me his party stories frequently. He did finally settle down and was saved in 1994. He always tells people he lost most of his friends and half his vocabulary when this happened.

Kevin's life was drastically altered when he became a paraplegic in January of 1998. He had an aneurysm on his descending aorta and due to the length of the surgery to correct this he became paralyzed. He went on to complete school in 2008 and became a social worker, where he then went on to work at a hospital...and met me!... And the rest is history...

KEVIN & MARIAH

We were married on quite possibly the coldest October day there ever was...October 4, 2014. The first few weeks were not the easiest but by December we were ready to start trying for that child we both felt confident belonged to us. I stopped my birth control right around Christmas that year and we began dreaming about the fun we would have the following Christmas with a little stub running around. I was confident this would be an easy feat, every month I convinced myself I was pregnant even though the odds of that were approximately 1 in 1,000,000,000. Due to Kevin's paraplegia, we obviously could not try for a child in the traditional rip your clothes off, spur of the moment, backseat kind of passion but there were some low-level interventions we attempted at home without the assistance of medical technology. As time went on and without success, it became obvious that this would not be the easiest thing we ever did...but we had no idea the journey that was about to begin.

Facebook post-March 1, 2014

"Trials are intended to make us think, to wean us from the world, to send us to the Bible, to drive us to our knees."

EVANSVILLE SEPTEMBER 2015

The fertility clinic is an interesting experience. Let me set this up for you because I'm convinced that they are all the same. Flowered carpet, plastic-covered chairs, HGTV on the tv and the most awkward waiting room silence you've ever experienced. The first visit to Boston IVF was a whirlwind of information and only slightly invasive. When we went over the statistics, I realized more so in my life than ever before that babies and pregnancy are a miracle! Dr. Griffin told us that even if everything works perfectly couples only have a 25% chance of getting pregnant with each cycle...so factor in the fact that I have polycystic ovarian syndrome and erratic cycles and Kevin is paralyzed below the waist and you can imagine our odds. We reviewed all kinds of family history and developed a plan to see a specialty urologist and attempt an IUI in the future. This begins major IVF lesson # 1...It is SLOW and you better be prepared to WAIT! Waiting is so so so hard, but I feel like waiting is where the boys are separated from the men (or girls separated from the women). The Bible is full of waiting. Noah had to wait for the flood, Lazarus had to wait to be raised from the dead, Moses had to wait to get out of Egypt and Abraham had to wait for a son. The waiting though...the waiting taught me lessons the outcome never could have.

The next few weeks and months were filled with multiple tests and appointments. I had to undergo some testing including bloodwork and something called a hysterosalpingogram (HSG) which is a test where they shoot dye up your hoohaa to make sure that it flows correctly through your fallopian tubes and there are no blockages. I tried to come up with some clever name for this that uses HSG but all I could come up with is THE MOST PAINFUL THING I HAD EXPERIENCED PRIOR TO LABOR!

When the nurse scheduled this test for me she told me it may be slightly uncomfortable and that I might want to take some ibuprofen prior to coming for the appointment. Understatement of the year. Up to this point, I hadn't had many procedures done "down there" so to strip off in a sterile room with an x-ray machine and have them shoot dye into my uterus was pretty humiliating. The first time they put the dye in it wasn't so bad and then Dr. Griffin said we have to do that again, we didn't get it in the right spot...the second time around the tears started flowing, the nurse looked over and said we got the right place this time. I drove myself to Evansville that day and I bet I cried halfway home. I was hurting and I was mad. Mad that I had to do this, Mad that it hurt so bad, and Mad that I couldn't make a baby like everyone else.

Kevin and I went to see a specialty urologist in St. Louis. Now I have never been to an abortion clinic but I would venture to say that they probably look like this office. The doctor was nice... you know for the teenager that he appeared to be. He reviewed our options. 1) It was possible that we would not need medical intervention to get Kevin's swimmers, but he would have to have a test at the IVF clinic to determine that. 2) There was what the medical clinic would call a non-invasive procedure (Kevin would likely disagree) to get the swimmers; however, this doctor had never performed it, but he would be willing to try or 3) There was a pretty invasive procedure they could use that would require an operating room and general anesthesia.

We returned to the fertility clinic for option number 1. That's when we got to experience the "little room" that everyone thinks of when they think about the male portion of the fertility clinic. It was just as awkward as everyone imagines!! The tv, the videos, the magazines, the plastic couch, the little cup you have to return when you're done and the awkward fact that you know people on the opposite side of the door can both hear you and know how long you've been in the room. Ultimately they thought it was possible that due to Kevin's paralysis his sperm was exiting through his urine, so we turned in a urine sample that day.

We had a return appointment scheduled, but it was changed to an over the phone situation. We were both off work that day in the fall of 2015. Kevin was working in the yard and I was stalking the phone. This was the appointment where they planned to review all our results. I was on pins and needles. When the phone rang I flagged Kevin down and we got some of the most important information of our lives on speakerphone right there in the garage. We were told that my egg levels looked appropriate, but Kevin's sperm count was nonexistent in his urine so we would need to proceed with further intervention. The doctor also told us that day that I carried a gene for fragile X syndrome, it was a recessive gene though and it was determined that my child would not be affected but that it was possible that my child's child may be affected someday.

Obviously, we did not desire to return to the teenage abortion clinic for the procedure he had never attempted before but would be willing to try so we were referred to a different specialist that was used to working with our IVF doctor.

LOUISVILLE—Part 1

Very important fact— We live in Southern Illinois and we observe daylight savings time…Louisville Kentucky does not…we learned this tidbit of information when we were an hour late for our first appointment in Louisville. When we did arrive, I realized we were not in Kansas anymore. This urology office was huge, the centralized waiting room probably had 100 seats. When we met Dr. Schrepferman, we were immediately impressed. He knew his stuff and it showed. Most doctors and nurses in our area are a little caught off guard by Kevin's paralysis; however, Dr. Schrepferman had worked at the Christopher Reeve center…He presented the same next 2 options as teenage doctor; however, instead of being willing to attempt option number 2—he had performed it countless times. We set up a plan to proceed with this option—the really good part about this doctor is that he had worked with Dr. Griffin multiple times so the 2 doctors would coordinate that. We left that office that day in high spirits!

The LION SLEEPER—NOVEMBER 2015

In November of 2015 on a typical Sunday, the sermon at our church was about preparing for your dream—we went to Wal-Mart after church to grab something quick for lunch and I made a detour to the baby department. I picked out a sleeper that day—a newborn sized green and blue striped sleeper with a lion on the front of it, a sleeper for the baby we would have someday. When we got home we hung the sleeper in our room—it would make a few moves (I will discuss them later), but for the most part, it hung on a knob on my dresser for 1,039 days before our baby wore it. This sleeper was the beginning of a big journey. I didn't realize it at the time—but the need to prepare for our baby would hold deeper meaning in the many months and years to come.

Facebook post-November 26, 2015: *"The Stubblefield thankful list of 2015, We are thankful for…#27) what we already know God is going to do for us and our family in 2016."*

Facebook post-December 13, 2015: *"Blessed is she who has believed that the Lord would fulfill His promises to her. Luke 1:45"*

VERY READY TO GET STARTED—IUI

Throughout this process, the waiting was the hardest part. We had sought help in September and Christmas rolled around with basically no progress. Christmas was hard…the previous Christmas was when we began "trying" for a baby and I was certain we would have one or at least would be pregnant by this Christmas and nothing…

In January of 2016, we were FINALLY ready to actually proceed with the baby-making. To complete the IUI I would begin medicine to produce increased eggs and when the timing was right we would travel to Louisville to the urologist to get Kevin's sperm and then back to Evansville for the procedure the following day.

As I would later learn an IUI is worlds easier than IVF. I began the oral meds for IUI and the subcutaneous shots in the stomach. After several days on the meds, I traveled to Evansville for an ultrasound where they decided I had produced enough of the appropriately sized eggs to proceed.

Kevin and I traveled to Evansville where we picked up the "retrieval kit" and checked into a hotel for the night. Very early the next morning Kevin and I traveled to Louisville for his procedure. Because of the timing of the procedures and the fact that the appointment could not be scheduled ahead of time and actually depended on my body, we had to arrive bright and early that day. In fact, we were the first appointment and we were going to be done with our appointment before the actual office hours began for the day. I was allowed to stay in the room while it was completed. While Kevin didn't exactly feel the procedure he did feel some uncomfortableness and I assure you his dignity and pride were hurt a little, but he sucked it up and did it for me. Now we had chosen this doctor's office over the abortion clinic type office because it seemed much more on the up and up; however, I have to tell you that morning was a bit sketchy. Kevin's procedure would take place in one room and the "results" would be taken to the room next door where a specialty "sperm doctor" would review the results right there to ensure the procedure was successful. We also had to bring a separate check that day and make it out directly to the "sperm reviewer." He must make interesting conversation when people ask what he does for a living. I nearly jumped for joy when we were told the procedure was successful. We loaded up with our "cooler" full of the goods and headed for Evansville.

We dropped the "boys" off at the fertility clinic and proceeded to the hotel to rest up for the next day. The next morning we arrived at Boston IVF and were called back into the room. I was so so sure this was the day I was going to become pregnant. Before they began the procedure we were told that while they did get sperm from Kevin the count was extremely low making the odds of this procedure working nearly impossible; however, since I had taken all the meds and we had the sperm we did we might as well proceed. It is pretty unromantic—"the turkey baster" method so to speak. The sperm was put in and I had to lay flat on my back for 15 minutes and then we were up and on our way home. We would have blood work done in about 2.5 weeks to see if it worked or not. That was it—on with normal life.

On the way home, we actually stopped at a used car lot to look at a truck Kevin had his eye on and would end up buying in the waiting period. The first vehicle we purchased together— probably not the smartest thing to do during the couple of weeks you should be stress-free—but life goes on…that's an interesting lesson throughout our entire infertility journey—life goes on— ALWAYS.

Some people choose to take home pregnancy tests while waiting for their lab work and some choose to wait (I call these people the strong ones). Kevin convinced me I should wait, which is what is recommended. I was beyond sure that this was going to work. I really wasn't that nervous and was able to forgo the testing because of how sure I was. I thought this IUI was the big mountain we had to climb—we would do this one round and we would get a baby, I probably have never been more wrong about anything in my whole life.

I actually had the pregnancy test blood work done at the local hospital and went to work. I waited for the phone call that I was sure would tell me I was pregnant. When the call came in that is not what the nurse on the other end of the phone told me. Instead, she told me my HCG level was 0 and I was not pregnant—I barely held it together on the phone—hung up and called Kevin. I then texted my mom and dad, the only message I really remember is the one to my dad. I told him it did not work and that I did not want to talk about it. I asked him to please comfort my mom because I knew she was as upset as me…and that was it—life went on—back to work I went.

Facebook post from January 17, 2016: *"It may be impossible, Nevertheless, God can do the impossible."*

Facebook post from January 30, 2016: *"It is well with my soul." "Faith in God includes Faith in his timing." "The pain that you've been feeling, can't compare to the joy that's coming. —Romans 8:18"*

What happens after IUI

I called the urologist office after the failed IUI to ask what they suggested we do next since the sperm count was not ideal. The doctor himself called me back one evening and to this day I still have the voicemail on my phone. He said that honestly with the results we had our best bet would be to go with the final more invasive option—freeze some higher quality sperm and proceed with IVF. I don't really remember exactly how I felt after that phone call—scared, nervous, mad, sad—all of the above.

IVF—Here we go

We returned to the doctor in Evansville to proceed with IVF—things went a little faster this time since we had already done the testing. A couple of really pertinent events stick out to me now as being ironic.

We met with the financial person from the fertility clinic to review our options for paying. When people tell you that IVF is expensive—believe them! Maddie ended up costing as much as your average house probably (obviously she is worth much more than a house). We had Kevin's insurance at this point so we would be paying for the entire IVF out of pocket. Kevin worked for a Catholic organization and since the Catholic faith does not believe in birth control or assisted fertility this was not something his insurance would cover. In the office that day we went over pricing—they had a deal if you wanted to sign up for 3 rounds of IVF—each got progressively cheaper—and I thought 3 times!! Who does this 3 times—we won't need that, we can't do that, we can't afford that! So we just paid for one—Oh how naïve I was!!

As we led up to beginning the first round I remember sitting in my car one day on my lunch break—I remember it like it was yesterday. The parking lot at my office kind of looked out over a big green field—I was eating lunch and watching YouTube videos about IVF. I watched one and the lady in the video said something about their 5th round of IVF and I thought to myself—Self: **5 TIMES!!! WHO DOES THIS 5 TIMES?!?! WHO CAN TOLERATE THIS 5 TIMES?!?! WHO CAN AFFORD THIS 5 TIMES?!?! I PROMISE I WILL NOT BE DOING THIS 5 TIMES!!!** What I didn't realize that day in the parking lot is the extent a mother will go to, to get to her child before she has even conceived, I didn't realize that when God plants a desire in your heart—you will get there no matter the bridges you have to cross—what I didn't realize is that it doesn't matter the cost financial, physical or emotional—once infertility sucks you in…you are in!

February 2016

Baby in a box—I have heard the box of meds that comes when you start an IVF cycle referred to as a baby in a box. It is a little overwhelming when you open that box—there are boxes and boxes of medicine. Medicine you take by mouth, medicine you inject in your stomach and medicine you inject intramuscularly in your butt (thigh). Some medicines need refrigerated, some don't, some have to thaw before you inject them, some you don't—some have to be given at a certain time and some don't. Truly, truly—it shows the extent a mother is willing to go through before she even conceives.

Prior to beginning meds, we returned to Louisville for the final procedure. We were beyond late for Kevin's appointment that day. It was just a weird day. We left in what should have been plenty of time and even remembered to account for the time difference this time around—but before we knew it we were running late—and then there was construction we had to detour around and then a wreck on the detour made us have to detour again. I called the office like 3 times that morning to say we were running late would they please wait for us…I think we got there like 2 hours late and still ended up waiting in the waiting room for like an hour. Come to find out the doctor had run late during surgery that morning and actually arrived at the office at the same time as us.

The procedure was much different this time. I was not allowed in there and sat in the hall in a chair. The nurse kept leaving the room and walking to a room across the hall with no update. I knew if this day was not successful we were done—this was our last chance to have Kevin's baby. When they finally did let me in the room they told me the procedure was much more difficult then they suspected it would be and if we ever needed more they would have to perform the procedure in a hospital under general anesthesia. Kevin never really let on but I imagine the procedure was pretty uncomfortable. We left that day with 12 vials of Kevin's sperm. That doesn't really mean a lot to me—ultimately we would use a technique that only required the amount of sperm per each of my eggs which would be 45. I don't know how many sperm per vial they retrieved but I know we had enough. We took a picture that day with the doctor and it would be the last time we saw him.

On February 27, 2016, I began the shots for our first IVF cycle. I wrote in a journal the next night—I wrote that I believed with my whole heart this cycle would result in my baby. That is my unwavering belief, my stupidity or my unwavering naivety—take your pick—that is present throughout this journey. No matter how many times we failed, I still believed success was right around the corner.

IVF was VERY, VERY, VERY different than IUI when it came to the medications and shots. For IVF I would have to take an intramuscular (IM) shot every night in the butt (thigh). Kevin would have to learn to give them to me. My dad was diagnosed with multiple sclerosis several years prior to this and had begun taking an IM shot weekly—his advice to me was to say the Lord's prayer while I was getting the shot to take my mind off of it, and that is what I did that night and every night after—I wrote in my journal that Kevin did not do a great job with that first shot but he was trying and that was a big deal for him.

I ended my journal entry with this quote that night… *"The important thing in life is not the triumph, but the struggle."*— Oh how true that statement would become in the years that followed.

You return to the fertility clinic approximately every other or every 2-3 days while taking IVF meds to get the lovely vaginal ultrasound and lab work. Some trips I took early in the morning and returned to work after and some I took the day off for. The first two trips of this cycle were taken early in the morning before work and were taken with my dad. He drove me the first time—I ran in for my lab work and hoohaa look and then we went to eat at IHOP—about 2 days later he took me again this time we ate lunch at Moe's on the way home—these would be the only 2 trips my dad would be a part of and I will forever cherish them. I know without a shadow of a doubt that he would have made 100 more trips with me if he could have.

Journal entry from March 5, 2016: *"Jesus replied, You do not realize now what I am doing, but later you will understand.— John 13:7. I know that YOU can only come from a certain egg and certain sperm and God was giving us YOU. Talk to you later, Love Mom"*

EGG RETRIEVAL

When the decision was finally made that we were ready for egg retrieval we traveled to Evansville. We went the night before and stayed in a hotel to be ready to go the next morning. Egg retrieval was relatively uneventful. When I woke up from the procedure Dr. Griffin came in to inform me how the procedure went. Unfortunately, he was only able to retrieve 2 eggs that day—this is extremely rare—generally multiple eggs are, somewhere more around 15 or 20. They would go ahead and proceed with the fertilization and go from there. We used a technique called ICSI which is where one sperm is injected into each egg rather than just mixing them together. Talk about nerve-wracking to leave your "babies" in a different state and wait for a phone call to hear about their "survival." We returned home and I rested that day.

The following day on a Sunday we awaited the call to tell us how many eggs fertilized. We were beyond naïve at this point and were so excited to hear. I had my phone on vibrate in church and when it went off I couldn't get outside fast enough. The nurse reported that BOTH eggs had fertilized and were growing—we would proceed with a day 3 transfer—she gave me all the instructions and we hung up. Kevin and I were so excited. I would later look back on this experience and know that it was terrible news to only get 2 eggs and it is not good to do a 3-day transfer... our odds were terrible, but we had no idea we were so excited. We went to lunch that day with one of Kevin's friends and Kevin told them what was going on—the first person aside from family that we told.

The next morning we headed in for PUPO day (Pregnant until proven otherwise). When you go in for implantation you have to drink 48-60 oz of water one hour before the transfer. About an hour before our appointment we stopped at the rest stop so I could pee and began drinking the water. I hate water—especially 60 oz. at a time but I downed it by the time we got there. We went in for the transfer—both got suited up in our hats and booties and the whole nine yards. Dr. Griffin came in to report on our embryos. He reported that one really didn't look good and had kind of stopped growing but they would implant it anyway and the other looked good. We went back to the room—I laid down spread eagle on the table which I would get used to and then they proceeded to press on my bladder with an ultrasound wand—I am convinced this part is to distract you from the entire process so that all you can think about is your need to pee (it is really to get your uterus in a good position to see, but I am not convinced). In went the two embryos—we watched on the screen and that was that. They let me off the table and we were released. First stop…bathroom—and as bad as I needed to pee when I got in the bathroom to do it, I couldn't—what if I peed them out?!?! (I know impossible, but trust me your mind goes there).

Last time's lack of testing was a no go for me from now on. I needed to be prepared for whatever news was coming. So about 3 days later I began the pee on a stick marathon. Anyone that has done infertility treatments knows what I'm talking about. The buy 2 or 3 pregnancy tests from a store about every other day to stock up and begin the marathon of peeing on a stick…but just to see nothing...ultimately the day before Easter we confirmed with lab work that this round was unsuccessful.

Journal entry for April 3, 2016: *"My heart broke into a million pieces with that phone call. Many tears fell over the next several days. Your dad was so strong for me. I'll never forget how he held me as I sobbed that night, he has been my rock. We are now discussing newborn adoption and have a phone interview set up. I'm scared and confused—but what I know for certain is that one day we will have YOU. I just don't know how you will get here. I promise to pray for you every day—however, you become. I love you so much already and will do whatever it takes to bring you home. For now, we will keep on keeping on until we get you. —Love Mom"*

ADOPTION

Adoption is something we had discussed before and Kevin was all for it but to be honest I was not all in. I wanted MINE and KEVIN's baby—I wanted to decide who the baby looked like, I wanted to be pregnant, I wanted to breastfeed a baby, I wanted to give Kevin the gift of flesh of his flesh. I didn't want someone else's baby. I understand that those are selfish wants but at this point in the journey, they were 100% true—but I was desperate for A BABY anyway that had to happen.

In April of 2016 I found myself in a place I never ever thought I would be. I thought IVF would be one and done—we had now done it and we were in no better place than we were before. We were not successful and we had no eggs in the freezer.

Facebook post from April 11, 2016: *"The Lord will never fail you. Just relax and keep praying."*

On April 13, 2016, we completed an interview with a newborn adoption agency. We learned many things that night, including the cost of newborn adoption which is actually more than a round of IVF. We learned the process to go through for a home study and we learned that honestly, the adoption process is just as iffy as the IVF process. On April 15, 2016, we got a phone call telling us we were accepted by Angel Adoption Agency and would need to decide whether we wished to proceed with them and if we did we needed to send them thousands of dollars.

In April of 2016, we also met with Dr. Griffin again to discuss the outcome of our previous attempt and the next steps he recommended. He told us that obviously, the cycle was not ideal. He discussed the medication changes he would make if we chose to proceed again. He also told us that day that after 3 egg retrievals if someone has no successful pregnancies he would not do anymore, but he counted our first as more of a half try due to my poor response to the meds. I had to humble my thoughts from before and discuss with the financial department if it was too late to sign up for the deal where you get a deal on multiple IVF trials. I never ever in a million years thought we would do this again and yet here we were with a huge decision to make. We could only afford to go one way (really we couldn't afford it, we would end up remortgaging our home in order to pay for our choice).

Journal entry from April 15, 2016: *"Today we got the news—Angel Adoption accepted us!! I am so excited. Your dad is a little leery but he will be on board soon enough! ...One more thing I don't want to forget—your Grandpa was so excited today when I told him. He practically jumped through the phone. We all love you so much!!—Love Mom"*

Facebook post from April 20, 2016: *"...Some events of the past year have made me realize how much my parents must miss him (my brother), I can't even imagine. Plainly said life sucks sometimes but in the eye of the storm, Jesus is still in control...ALWAYS".*

Facebook post from April 24, 2016: *"Joseph waited 13 years. Abraham waited 25 years. Moses waited 40 years. Jesus waited 30 years. If God is making you wait, you're in good company."*

I honestly don't remember exactly when or why we made our decision but ultimately we decided to turn down Angel Adoption and plan to proceed with another round of IVF in June of 2016.

SEE YOU ON THE OTHER SIDE

The first week of May 2016 I was the luckiest girl on the planet. I got to take a vacation to my most favorite place on Earth with my most favorite people on Earth! Kevin, myself and my mom and dad took a trip to Yellowstone National Park. It was Kevin's first time on a plane and first time to Yellowstone. We were all so excited.

So many times on that trip we joked about seeing each other on the other side. I remember when we went through security the very first time I said to my parents see you on the other side because Kevin and I would be slower, that became our running joke for the trip.

My dad's health was not the best and he had a few "episodes" of shortness of breath and feeling bad during the trip but overall we had a great time. We stopped to fill up the rental car with gas right before returning to the airport. My dad pumped the gas and went in to pay. The other 3 of us were waiting in the car when a firetruck pulled up with the lights on—I distinctly remember us joking about them really needing gas to stop on their way to a call—the medics got out and were putting gloves on to go inside—that's when my mom began to worry about my dad—she went in to check on him and when she didn't promptly return I went in. My dad had passed out in the bathroom and they were taking him to the hospital—as they were wheeling him out on the gurney he was talking and looked fine—he was not happy about going to the hospital. He and my mom insisted that Kevin

22

and I go on to the airport and fly home. They were certain they would be following that evening or the next day. Leaving that day is quite possibly one of the biggest regrets of my life.

Kevin and I proceeded to the airport. I was able to talk to my dad on the phone—he sounded great and said he was feeling fine. We boarded the plane and flew to our first stop. When we got off the plane we called to check and everything was still going well. They were running tests and checking him out but everything was fine. Kevin and I went to the food court to get lunch—as we were eating I got the call from my mom that my dad had coded and they were performing CPR. After several phone calls, it was determined I would fly back to Wyoming and Kevin would return home. They were able to resuscitate my dad and I proceeded to book my flight back. Kevin boarded his plane, I still had a couple of hours to wait for my flight. That was one of the hardest things I have endured—is watching half my heart return to Illinois and know the other half was hanging in limbo in Wyoming and I was stuck in the middle completely unable to get to either one of them. I never got off the phone and never sat down in that two-hour wait. I called anyone and everyone to keep from having to sit in silence. I had talked to my mom a couple of times and she told me they were working on him and that if they got him stabilized he would be flown to a bigger hospital. I was so scared.

That was the longest plane ride of my life—my phone had to be off and I was completely out of contact with everyone. The lady sitting next to me ultimately offered me a ride to the hospital when we landed. I spent that entire flight praying for my dad to be alive when I got to the hospital and I believed with every fiber of my being that he would be. When we got off the plane I had a voicemail from my mom saying she would likely be unable to answer the phone and she would see me when I got there.

The kind woman and her husband drove me to the hospital that night—it was probably 10 or 11 o'clock. I walked in and told them who I was looking for. It was a small hospital and the receptionist started to walk me to my mom. I asked her if my dad was alive—she responded that she would let me talk to my mom first. I distinctly remember my response "I work in a hospital, I know what that means". My dad died in Wyoming that night. He suffered from a heart arrhythmia and ultimately was unable to be resuscitated. Getting home and getting my dad's body home was surreal.

I distinctly remember when we arrived home that night. Kevin, our preacher and my Grandpa came to greet us on the porch. My mom went straight to hug her dad and I went straight to hug my husband. We both went straight to the person the other one of us no longer had—that has always stuck out to me. I remember looking over Kevin's shoulder as I was hugging him and seeing our preacher's face—it had a distinct look of sadness, of grief, of unbelief—I remember that distinct look and I would see the exact one again later that year.

I will forever miss the fact that my dad was unable to be a Grandpa and I will forever miss my dad. The fact that he was not alive that night when I got to the hospital despite my prayers has never deterred me from praying or believing then in the power of prayer.

Journal entry from May 12, 2016: *"Your Grandpa died. We decided to proceed in June Anyway."*—That was my last journal entry.

TAKE TWO

In June of 2016, we began round two of IVF. I remember being worried about starting back again so soon after losing my dad. I had to start oral meds the week after his death and Kevin and I did question whether we should proceed at that time. One of my very best friends said something that ultimately influenced my decision. She said to me " He is no more or less gone whenever you do it if this is what you want you need to get it."

I felt like a pro this time around. I knew how the shots worked, they were old hat, I knew about the meds and I knew about the many, many trips for lab work and ultrasounds. They used the same vein every time for my labs—it worked like a charm—"easy stick." I always joked that it knew what its job was. From the lab draw chair in the fertility clinic, you can see the "footprint" wall. Babies who were a product of this clinic had their footprint on the wall with their name and date of birth. I stared that wall down during so many blood draws. At the time I had the name memorized of the ones I could see.

This time we had success!! Twenty-three eggs were retrieved. I remember returning to work the next day which was likely a mistake. I distinctly remember sitting in my car after seeing a home health patient…I was so sore. Five of the eggs were viable and we ultimately ended up transferring two eggs.

Commence pee on a stick marathon again…and then on June 29, 2016 something new happened…that stick, it had two lines.

That is something I never ever thought I would see. When I got the phone call about the lab work it wasn't good news but I suppose it wasn't bad news either. My HCG level was 49…they like to see it around 100 at this point; however, anything over 5 is considered pregnant. I was pregnant!! And that is when we did what Kevin says we should never do…we let our highs get too high. They checked the level two days later to make sure it was doubling. I remember we were in the checkout line at Lowe's getting stain for our deck when the doctor's office called. When they gave me the results it did not double but it rose by 75% so we proceeded. They did one more lab draw and this time the number did double and so we waited about a week for the ultrasound.

At the first ultrasound, they found the gestational sac in my uterus, which erased fear number one of a possible ectopic pregnancy, they did not, however, find a heartbeat. Dr. Griffin told us that it was possible that it was just too early to see the heartbeat but it was also possible that it was not developing appropriately. He suggested we wait a few more days and have another ultrasound now that we knew it was not ectopic—so that is what we did. On July 25, 2016, we returned for the next ultrasound. No heartbeat was found. Dr. Griffin called me into his office after the ultrasound and we had to make some decisions. He presented my options. I could stop the meds and wait for a miscarriage to naturally happen; however, no one knew how long that may take, we could schedule a D & C to remove the pregnancy or he could prescribe a medication to induce the miscarriage. I remember asking if he was 100% sure this was not a viable pregnancy. I honestly didn't think he would be willing to answer that question—it is rare for doctors to admit they are 100% sure of anything. His answer to me was that he was 100% sure, but he was willing to wait as long as I wanted and to perform another ultrasound so that I could be 100% sure. That was good enough for me. I decided that I didn't want to start having a miscarriage while I was at work and there was no need for the D & C so we decided on the methotrexate to induce the miscarriage.

I waited until the weekend to use the medicine so that I could be at home in a controlled environment when it started. The methotrexate had to be inserted vaginally and the bleeding was expected to start a few hours later. Kevin had to work that day—after he left my grandparents stopped by—they knew to an extent what was happening. The only thing I remember about our conversation was that I questioned the "fairness" of the world—which was such a naïve thing to think or question. The world obviously is not fair. I remember talking about people who have one night stands and end up pregnant and contemplating abortion yet go on to have healthy babies. I remember asking my Grandpa why they got to have a baby when they didn't even want one and thought about killing theirs and I didn't get to have one…and I remember his answer he just shook his head and told me he didn't know.

When they left I "took" the medicine—well I don't know if took is the right word—I "inserted" the medicine and went to sulk on the couch. I don't remember exactly but I would guess probably 20 or 30 minutes later the pain and the bleeding started. I don't remember a lot about that day, I just remember the pain and the clots…lots and lots of clots. I don't know when I passed the "baby". They had given me a collection cup to search through the clots and find the fetal tissue to send for a biopsy but Dr. Griffin told us that the results would likely not assist in any further attempts so we opted not to do that. I also remember thinking about the irony of spending literally thousands of dollars to "build up" your uterine lining just to get to feel the pain and deal with the blood of passing all of the lining.

Facebook post from August 3, 2016: *"I know I often need a reminder and maybe someone else out there does too. It sometimes feels like God can't hear us or isn't listening...but we must remember he is ALWAYS in control. He is with us always, and if he chooses not to move a mountain for us...at least we will know we have a climbing partner. For God has said I will never fail you. I will never abandon you. —Hebrews 13:5"*

"The strongest people are not those who show strength in front of us, but those who win battles we know nothing about"

HERE WE GO AGAIN

〜✦〜

Waiting…waiting…waiting. If I had to choose one word to describe IVF, waiting would quite possibly be it. We were ready to try again following the *miscarriage* in July but due to a variety of reasons, it would be November before we could try again.

Facebook post from August 27, 2016: *"Best battle plan against the enemy is often: I'm still standing!"*

September 22, 2016: *I posted an article on Facebook titled 'Why God Took So Long TO Give Me A Baby'—"Good read. Could also be said about many other things in life…whatever you are waiting for, God is in control of and is waiting until the right time. The waiting is so so so hard, rest assured God has not forgotten and when you get it, the wait won't even matter anymore. "Having patiently endured, he received the promise." –Hebrews 6:15"*

October 16, 2016: *"The pain that you've been feeling, can't compare to the joy that's coming. –Romans 8:18"*

November 6, 2016: *"When you go through deep waters, I will be with you. –Isaiah 43:2"*

Shortly before Thanksgiving of 2016, one of the people I worked very closely with at work had a baby. She too had struggled with having this baby (her 2nd child) for different reasons but still, it was a struggle for her. I remember about a year before that we had gone to lunch and each discussed our struggles to have a baby and agreed to pray for each other, and here she was getting exactly what she wanted, it would be a lie to say that was easy for me. See that's something that is truly difficult for people who have never experienced infertility to understand, it is possible to be happy for someone, but also be sad for yourself and to be happy for someone but to skip the baby shower out of self-preservation. Infertility is tricky ground.

November 24, 2016: I posted my 'thankful list for the year' 2) My husband who has been my rock on more than one occasion this year and for his faith that is far greater than mine. 10) Despite the sadness of this year, I still have hope in Jesus Christ. 12) Even in the eye of the storm, Jesus is still in control. 15) Modern medicine, that helps to provide choices and options. 23) Things being as well with me and my family as they are. 24) The mindset to continue to be thankful!!

In November of 2016, we proceeded with another transfer. 2 more embryos were implanted in me. Pee on a stick marathon here we come....positive again! This time, however, we kept our highs in check. The first blood draw...great numbers, the second blood draw...numbers more than doubled. We were starting to get somewhat excited but trying to keep our emotions in check, but surely something bad wouldn't happen twice in a row. My mom and I were planning to leave for a vacation to the Smokey Mountains the morning of the third blood draw when I went to the bathroom that morning and wiped there was some spotting on the toilet paper and I was convinced it was over. We went to the doctor's office and had my blood drawn then proceeded with our trip. We were on the road when the doctor's office called with the news...the numbers...had skyrocketed! They were great!!!

They scheduled one more blood draw for when I returned from my vacation. I questioned the bleeding at they said that some women just have spotting throughout their pregnancy and maybe I was just going to be one of those women, but according to my numbers which is all we could go off of right now everything looked great. So we proceeded through the vacation, hindered slightly by the big wildfire that shut Gatlinburg down. Every time I went to the bathroom I checked the toilet paper and then gave my mom a rundown when I came out. The spotting slowed down and came and went from day to day.

DECEMBER 6, 2016

We had returned from vacation, I was headed back to work but went to the doctor's office for bloodwork first. When they called with the numbers they were fantastic...super high, everything was just as it should be. We discussed the spotting again and again they said that it just happens to some women and so I went on with work. I remember when the pain started...I was doing a wheelchair evaluation and just couldn't quite get comfortable sitting on the mat next to the patient. There was a nagging sensation at the top of my left hip, but if I shifted just right I could relieve it. When I finished the evaluation I called Dr. Griffin's office, the nurse questioned my pain symptoms and gave me some possibilities of what could be causing it—she reviewed my numbers and again discussed how great they looked and said that we really had nothing else to go off of for another week or so until they could see something on the ultrasound. So I went back to work.

The pain gradually got a little worse throughout the day. I remember my last patient of the day that day was a home health patient and I was fine as long as I was up walking around the house with her and standing, but when I was sitting in the car at the end to finish my note I remember I couldn't get comfortable. Driving home I could not hold still the pain was increasing. I called Kevin and my mom. Kevin had to work late that night so my mom came over to be with me. The pain eased some but I went ahead and called the doctor's office on-call number. I got to talk to Dr. Griffin himself who said that really the only thing to be concerned about would be an ectopic pregnancy but that my numbers pretty much ruled that out, he told me to take some ibuprofen and see if it eased the pain and said that if it worsened I should go to the ER.

My mom got there and offered to cook me supper but I really didn't have an appetite. I remember she made me chicken noodle soup and I only ate about 4 or 5 bites (isn't it weird how seemingly normal everyday activities can later stick in your mind after the day becomes significant?). She and I discussed the possibility of appendicitis, but by then the ibuprofen was kicking in and I felt a little better and Kevin was home. I went to lay on the couch and my mom went home. She went to talk to Kevin before she left and told him the two main things we were worried about and why they were so serious. After a while, I went to take a shower thinking the warm water would help. I googled the symptoms of appendicitis and got pretty worried that may be what was wrong. After talking it over with Kevin we decided to go to the ER. We called my mom and she said she would meet us there.

They got us right in at the ER (Kevin and my mom both worked at that hospital—that always helps). The doctor went over that ectopic was their first concern so they would do an ultrasound. As the ultrasound technician was wheeling me back for the ultrasound I remember asking if she would tell me what she saw even though they weren't supposed to. She implied that she would "cheat" a little and tell me what she saw. We got to the room and we did the ole vaginal ultrasound…she was very quiet. After a few minutes, I asked what she was seeing and she told me she would rather the doctor go over the results with me, and that's when I knew…something was wrong. I returned to the ER room and the doctor came in to tell us that it was in fact an ectopic pregnancy…we all cried, all three of us. We would have to proceed with surgery that night to remove the ectopic since it was already leaking blood and causing pain. The bleeding just got worse as the night went on. Due to another case being worked on we had to wait quite a while in the ER.

When I woke up from surgery and the doctor came in to talk to me, he informed me that I actually had a pregnancy in each of my tubes, a bilateral ectopic pregnancy (I know, I know it is super rare!). He was able to remove one from the tube and sew the tube back up, but the other had already started to burst so he had to remove the whole tube. After I woke up in recovery we proceeded up to a room where I would stay for several hours before going home. There are 2 distinct things I remember about that day.

1. When we got to the room a nurse that I had worked very closely with was my nurse. She had to examine me… which involved raising my gown and pulling the pad from between my legs to see how much I was bleeding and at that moment I lost all my dignity. Here I had failed at another pregnancy and someone was assessing the pad between my legs.

2. I had fallen asleep shortly after getting to the room and when I woke up I saw our preacher standing in front of my bed…and there was that face again. The one I saw in May the face of severe pity, the look of I can't believe your life is this bad…we made eye contact and we both just shook our heads… how on earth was this happening?

We returned home and had a follow up with Dr. Griffin. He could not believe this happened. He said he had no explanation for it, because even if the catheter had been in the wrong place when implanting the embryos that would only explain one ectopic, not one in each tube. We would proceed with another transfer, but of course, we would need to wait a month or so. I also had a follow up with Dr. Albright the one who performed the surgery, when I saw him that's when I realized we were now cool. He showed me pictures they had taken of my tubes. The one they had to remove you really couldn't tell much, it was starting to separate which is why I had the pain, the other tube; however, they were able to just cut open and remove the embryo—I could see the outline of the embryo—of course, it didn't look exactly like a baby, but I could see the outline— where the head and the spine were. The hospital I went to has a program where you can see your chart online—I would later read the ultrasound report from that night and learn that the baby I could see the outline of actually had a heartbeat that night. It was very low obviously and incompatible with life…but it had a beating heart…just growing in the wrong place. We were the couple with a weird medical situation, he said he had never seen a bilateral ectopic before. So we were cool but still childless.

Facebook post-December 10, 2016: *"Jesus answered and said to him, What I am doing, you do not understand now, but you will understand later. –John 13:7"*

December 21, 2016: *"The pain that you've been feeling, can't compare to the joy that's coming. –Romans 8:18"*

December 31, 2016: *"2016, was not a good year, in fact, I'll venture to say it was the worst year of my life; however, that being said I know my year was 100 times better than some people's year and for that I am thankful. Also in saying that it does not mean 2016 was without some good times, including a family vacation, a mom and* *daughter vacation, a happy and healthy husband and mom, a job that I enjoy (most of the time) and many other blessings that I don't ever want to take for granted. Each year is but a blip in the scheme of forever, but tonight I have no hesitation in saying sayonara 2016, hit the road jack, don't let the door hit you on the way out. Tomorrow is a fresh start and I'm ready for it, 2017 is going to be a good year!"*

AND AGAIN...

Again, the waiting, it was February before we could try again. There was some internal healing that had to take place from my surgery and it always took a while to get cycles lined up but in February we were ready to go. It was our last egg...just one left, (my naivety kicked in again) I remember thinking, this was God's plan all along. We would not have any embryos left we had to make hard decisions about and we wouldn't end up with a bunch of kids, it was perfect I was sure it was going to work. We proceeded with the meds, the shots, the multiple appointments to decide when we were ready and then we did another transfer our fourth. It was oddly not as exciting by now.

One of the girls I work with started IVF at this time also. I remember her texting me and using code, saying she was having a few medical procedures done that she may need a couple of days off for but that she was told she could resume "normal" activities just taking it easy, and I knew exactly what she was doing. I really struggled with whether or not to say anything but I ultimately did and we immediately bonded over our shared struggle. We were just about a week or two apart in the process. She found out she was pregnant about the time I was going in for my transfer.

The pee on a stick marathon began again (I really should have taken stock out in pregnancy tests). There was the line, and it was getting darker, but then we had been here before. When I got the call with the results the number was right where it should be 170!!! They hope for anything over 100 at this point and since there was only one this time it could not be the same problem as last time. I knew it, this last one was going to be it! I called my newfound IVF friend from work and we laughed about how our employer was going to have a hard time since we would both be on maternity leave at the same time. We got that lab work on a Thursday so it was going to be Monday before they did it again. By Saturday the peeing on a stick was not going well. The line was definitely getting lighter. I took multiple pictures and made Kevin and my mom compare them all. Kevin tried to reassure me that I was overthinking it all. I googled everything under the sun, tried to convince myself maybe I had drunk more and diluted the urine, maybe I didn't take them at the right time, maybe it was the dye in the tests, but truthfully in my heart, I knew it wasn't working. When I got my lab work done on Monday they confirmed the number had fallen, again I tried to convince myself that maybe it had separated into twins and one failed and it would go back up...but it was over this cycle had failed also. I remember sending a message to the girl from work, it said I guess November won't be so bad for our bosses after all. We were out of frozen embryos and still childless.

Facebook post-March 21, 2017: *I posted an article about the loss of a baby, "A good article. Loss of any kind is so hard...and sometimes makes us long to be in heaven too, but we must remember that all things work for the good of those that love him, and whatever is happening it is part of the plan. I know this, I will have a great reunion waiting for me in heaven and I can't wait. But, that is not for now, for now, I'm on Earth and I'm going to do my best to live until I die!"*

I NEVER THOUGHT WE WOULD DO THIS MORE THAN ONCE

Remember that video I watched of the people that did IVF 5 times and I thought they were crazy, remember when I thought it was crazy to sign up for the multiple IVF discount. Here we were having to make a choice. Do we do this again?? Or remain childless?? IVF is stressful, IVF is painful, IVF is emotionally draining, it is hard to work and arrange appointments, but most of all IVF is expensive!! In order to be able to do IVF again, we would need to come up with the money to pay for it. See that's the thing they require the money upfront.

We ended up remortgaging our house to get the funds, we borrowed from my parents and we shuffled insurances. In for a penny (or millions and billions of pennies) in for a pound, we were doing this again. We were crazy, we were insane, we had terrible odds, but we were faithful and we wanted a baby.

Facebook post-April 19, 2017: *"Warning this is a long post, but I felt like it all needed to be said. I know I use this picture every year, but it's one of my favorites, this is how I choose to remember him. 12 years ago tomorrow (it seems unreal that it has been that long, very soon he will have been gone longer than I had him here)this guy left this world to go "home". To be honest, it's hard to explain but my life is not altered every day because he is gone, because honestly the majority of "my life" has happened since he left, but the idea of him I miss so much, a big brother to have over for dinner, his wife that could* *have been my friend, his children that could have been my nieces and nephews, his comfort when dad went to heaven this year, but my mom...my heart breaks for her because I cannot imagine how much her heart longs for him to be here. This has been a year like no other for sure, but it has made me think a lot and I don't want this to be a sad, woe is me post because you know what, this world is not what it was intended to be, it is full of pain and sorrow (and though sometimes it feels like it's only my pain and sorrow, the truth is EVERYONE has pain and sorrow), but one day...oh one day we're going HOME where there are streets of gold and no sadness!!! So tomorrow I'll remember him a little extra and smile when I think about the reunion that has taken place this year when N and C knife traders was reunited! But I will not let the sadness linger or get stuck in it, because I have some living left to do before I go "home" too, see you later bub!!"*

In April of 2017, we did another round of drugs and retrieved 20 eggs, 4 of which survived and became viable. This round was much rougher on me. The drugs made me a little sicker, I was much, much sorer for several days after the retrieval. I don't really know what the difference was, except I was one year older and the excitement was gone. It was no longer this exciting journey that I was sure was going to get us a baby. We had done ALL of this before with terrible outcomes. Nurses at the fertility were starting to leave, we had been there longer than a lot of the staff, it just wasn't fun and I'll be honest I was sad. This hadn't worked before and this time we ended up with FEWER embryos, but the number doesn't matter, because it truly only takes one.

After retrieval, we proceeded with implantation and implanted 2 embryos...you know the routine by now. Pee on a stick, over and over and over again, this time we didn't get good numbers once or twice, we got GREAT numbers every time they tested. This was uncharted territory—we had never been here before.

NEW TERRITORY

On May 15, 2017, I went for the first ultrasound my mom drove me, I'm sure people will question why Kevin didn't go, but truthfully at this point, we had had so many appointments he couldn't possibly have missed work for them all, my job was much more flexible than his, and in all honesty, we had come to expect the worst and didn't see the need in getting our highs too high. I remember thinking about letting my mom come in the room with me, but it is a little awkward—these aren't the over-the-stomach ultrasounds if you know what I mean. Most of all; however, I didn't want her to be in the room because I was afraid it was going to be bad news and my goal was ALWAYS to not cry in the doctor's office and I knew if the two of us were in there together neither of us could hold it together. So in I went.

Missy would end up being my favorite at the fertility clinic, I don't know if she was yet or if it would be later but ultimately she was my favorite. She did my ultrasound that day…then she said these words…there is the heartbeat 125 BPM and I remember like yesterday my exact words "I just took a deep breath for the first time in 2 years." She continued with the ultrasound and Dr. Griffin came in to look at everything—everything looked great! Then they handed me the most precious picture I had ever been given, my baby with a beating heart safely nestled in my uterus where he belonged. On the way to the car, I called Kevin—I wanted him to be the first to hear and then I got in the car and showed the picture to my mom. And then I did it again…my highs got very high!

I was scheduled to go back for a follow-up ultrasound just to ensure that everything was ok the following week and in the meantime, Kevin and I had a trip planned to Texas. We took the vacation on cloud 9. We were visiting some old friends of Kevin's on that trip and he told them about the pregnancy and we showed off our picture all week. I was pregnant…for real! On that trip, I even experienced some very mild morning sickness and nausea and to be honest kind of enjoyed it. Our first day back from the trip we went for the follow-up ultrasound and this time Kevin came with me, and we heard the words again there is the heartbeat. 155 BPM this time, we got pictures of what looked like a tiny gummy bear. I remember the conversation between Dr. Griffin and Kevin—Dr. G: "It is very unlikely that anything would go wrong at this point" Kevin: "Don't say that doc, you know us, the weird stuff happens to us." Dr. Griffin laughed but said that really we were past the scary part. We were 9 weeks pregnant after trying so so so hard and failing so so so many times. We couldn't wait to tell the world. We took our gummy bear picture and cell phone recorded video of a beating heart and took pictures with Dr. Griffin and just like that, we were released to our OB.

We told the world that night. Both our moms came over we took pictures and made it official via Facebook.

Facebook post-May 24, 2017: *"Warning this is going to be a long post, but I promise the end is worth it, but don't skip to the end without reading the whole thing or you might miss a blessing…just like we would have. I have thought about this post for years!!! 2 years and 5 months to be exact. How would I put it on Facebook, first I thought a picture of Kam or a chalkboard announcement, then as the trying took months and we proceeded to specialists in Evansville and Louisville I thought about pictures of needles…but it progressed far* *beyond that and so I want to make this announcement by giving God the glory he deserves for being the giver of life!!! In February of 2016, Kevin and I underwent a procedure to get pregnant that was unsuccessful, so we proceeded with IVF the first round was done in March of 2016 and was also unsuccessful, we then decided to try again, in June of 2016, we underwent another round of IVF which sadly ended in a miscarriage at 7 weeks when the baby never developed a heartbeat, we did another round in December of 2016, which ended in a bilateral ectopic pregnancy with a baby in each tube, with emergency surgery and loss of 1 tube. We remained determined and tried again in February of 2017, which again resulted in a miscarriage. We decided to try one last time we both agreed this would be the last round…we don't know why God didn't move this mountain for us, but we do know he climbed it right beside us or we would never have made it. So so so many people have prayed for this baby and I will never be able to thank them enough. When I didn't know what to pray or couldn't pray anymore I am so thankful for those that filled the gap for me!! I would love to say my faith never wavered during this process but that would be a lie…there were times I'm not even sure I had the faith of a mustard seed, but I had faith and faith can move mountains!!! God is the giver of life and we give him all the praise and glory for this child!! We are beyond thankful and happy!!! While we firmly believe God made this baby, he used some people here to help set up the meeting and we are beyond thankful for them also, Boston IVF in Evansville and all their WONDERFUL staff, Dr. Griffin, and Dr. Schrepferman. I said all that to say baby Stubblefield is due January 2018."*

Our OB didn't want to see us until at least 11 weeks, so we just floated along for a couple of weeks. I would be lying if I said I didn't pee on a few sticks in those couple of weeks, doubting Thomas if you will.

Facebook post-June 10, 2017: I posted an article about a dog and an elephant getting pregnant at the same time but the elephant has to wait so much longer for its baby, and I wrote this. *"I have read this before, and I love it. Throughout this process, God and I have had many talks, and I told him when (not if, but when) he gave me a baby, I was going to make sure the world heard my story. I'm going to make sure the world knows what GOD can do. Before this is over I'm sure many of you will get tired of my postings and that's ok because if the message of faith and God's goodness reaches one new person every time it will have been worth it. When my baby hits the ground, the world will feel it!!! And for that I'm thankful!"*

The weekend before my first OB appointment I had some bleeding. It was a Friday night, and I panicked. I had immersed myself in the pregnancy world for multiple years and I have a degree in the medical field, so I knew there was nothing they could do even if I was having a miscarriage and still I panicked. I called the on-call number for Boston IVF and talked to Missy—she of course told me there was nothing they could do. She went over what to do if the bleeding got too heavy and tried to reassure me that bleeding didn't always mean miscarriage. The bleeding slacked off over the weekend and I had an appointment scheduled for Monday morning. When I went in for the appointment all I wanted was to see an ultrasound and see my baby, but we had to go through the whole rigmarole of medical history, vitals, blah, blah, blah. When the doctor finally came in to do the ultrasound he was quiet for too long—he was doing an over-the-belly ultrasound this time which was a new experience all in itself. When I couldn't take the quiet anymore I said there is no heartbeat is there? The doctor promptly apologized for taking so long and said that I shouldn't worry yet and then he found it. He wanted them to take a closer look so he sent me to the ultrasound room for the fun vaginal ultrasound. I remember when I got in there she made a big deal about leaving so I could get undressed but I told her don't bother, I was used to this.

She found the heartbeat no problem and said everything looked good with the baby. I had a small subchorionic hematoma. A collection of blood, she told me it was smaller than the baby and they really only ever worry about them if they get big. She told me I may pass the blood or my body may absorb it, but that overall everything looked good. The doctor gave me the option to come monthly like "typical" pregnant women or to come every other week if that would make me feel better—obviously that was my choice. So I left in good spirits that day.

Facebook post-June 17, 2017: *"A new reason to celebrate Father's day this year!! Some would say he's not a father yet but I disagree. He has had to work hard for this miracle too. He has driven a sleeping wife to many, many appointments, he has become an expert shot giver, he has dried countless tears, consoled a sad wife hyped up on hormones, encouraged when it seemed hopeless and prayed many many prayers. He is already an awesome dad and while he's technically a father to be this year I'm still celebrating him!!! Love you bunches, Kevin Stubblefield!"*

June 28, 2017

I was off work on the day of June 28th, 2017. I had a doctor's appointment first thing that morning and Kevin was going with me. I had had some spotting on and off but no terrible bleeding, I had been to the doctor one other time since that first appointment and everything looked good. I still had the subchorionic hematoma (SCH) but they kept saying it was smaller than the baby and would likely resolve. We had passed the 12-week mark and were feeling very confident. The doctor came in and talked to us then sent us to get an ultrasound. They started with the over the belly but decided they needed a few better pictures so we went with the ole internal again…oh boy. There was the regular ultrasound tech who I'm pretty sure was also a nurse and there was a student. The student inserted the ultrasound probe and I remember it being so uncomfortable, which was odd because I was so used to these, I had had so many and this was the worst. I remember Kevin asking if they could tell the sex of the baby and the experienced tech looked at the big screen, she explained that they couldn't be sure and they were going more based of the "angle of the dangle" than actual anatomy but that she thought boy definitely, I remember Kevin pumping his fist into the air, I remember the excitement and then I remember the silence. The experienced tech took over for the student because she wanted to see something better, I remember asking if something was wrong and she just kept avoiding my question. She told me to get dressed and went to talk to the doctor. We met the doctor in the hallway and I remember she said the bleed was right over my cervix now and I should expect some more bleeding and that they would see me again in 2 weeks but just for a regular appointment, not for a special ultrasound. To me, that seemed like we must be progressing, so Kevin went to work and I went to my mom's for the day. We were going to enjoy my day off relaxing and swimming. When I got to my mom's house she wasn't home yet, as I walked into the house I remember feeling something between my legs, I went to the bathroom and there was a lot of blood. I immediately called the doctor's office. It was a big office with multiple doctors and a call center so it was difficult to talk to anyone I had actually seen and kept leaving messages. I also remember calling a different OB office to try and get moved because I felt like I wasn't getting good service. They took my information and said they would call me back.

The bleeding continued throughout the day. I laid on my mom's couch all day long in hopes that if I lay still enough the bleeding would stop. I know—there is no science behind that and it was silly to think, but I didn't know what else to do. On my way home the doctor finally called me back. She asked about the bleeding—we went over how much, she asked about cramping and I told her I hadn't had any. She made an appointment for me to come in the next day and we hung up. Probably an hour or so later the cramping started. In my head, I knew what was happening but my heart didn't want to believe it. The bleeding and cramping continued that night until I couldn't sit still due to the pain. It was the worst pain of my entire life, it was at least 2 or 3x as bad as the ectopic pain. I told Kevin I knew the ER couldn't do anything but I needed to know what was happening and if it was bad then at least they could give me some pain medicine, and so we made our second trip to the ER for a failing pregnancy. As I was signing in at the triage desk I remember a nurse coming out to the desk, as I was explaining what was going on I felt a large clot pass between my legs and told the nurse I was having a problem. I wish I remembered that nurse's name because at that moment I feel like she chose me to take mercy on that night. She immediately took me back to a room and got me into a bed.

She went to talk to the doctor then promptly came back. She helped me get out of my pants which was just the beginning of a humiliating experience. I remember her taking the soggy pad out of my underwear and commenting that there were no large clots which was a good sign. She got me in the bed. The doctor quickly popped in and said he was ordering blood work and an ultrasound. I remember looking up at Kevin and mouthing "it's over" and he shook his head no as if to say just hold on, but I knew... it was my body, I knew what was happening. As the nurse went to leave I told her I passed another large clot, she looked between my legs and went into the hall. I heard her say to the doctor "she passed it." When she came back in I asked, "Did you say I passed it?" She nodded yes and scooped something up between my legs. I remember looking at Kevin and he was crying...I'm not sure I had ever seen him cry before. At some point on the way to the ER we had called my mom and she arrived. I looked up at her as she came into the room and said I lost the baby. She lost it, so did I and so did Kevin. The nurse came back in to help me get into those mesh underwear everyone talks so much about and I remember asking for pain medicine. It truly was the most painful thing I had ever felt. I truly believe it was labor pains. I remember standing in the ER room, Kevin had wheeled around the corner, I was standing over a chucks pad to catch the blood, the nurse was trying to wipe the blood from my legs and my mom was helping me get the underwear and pad on, it truly was a humbling experience. That nurse was so kind and she sopped up my blood.

I remember as I was getting back into bed I asked, "How much blood can a person lose and still be ok?" And her response, "A lot."

A woman that we went to church with was a nurse in the ER that night and she came in to bring me my pain medicine, I remember telling her through the sobbing and the tears that she could ignore the HIPPA rules and tell her family what happened because I didn't want to have to. At that moment it was hitting me that we had gone public and were now going to have to take it all back. We let our high get way, way too high.

The nurse came in to go over our options. We could send the "baby" to medical waste and just have it honored in a hospital-wide ceremony, or we could choose to handle the remains ourselves. Kevin didn't speak up about much that night but I remember him saying "it is our baby, we will take care of it." Actually, it turns out that if we kept "him" at the hospital it would be considered medical waste, but if we chose to handle the remains, it would have to go through a funeral home. The nurse asked if we wanted to see the baby and I said yes.

She brought in this perfectly formed little boy. He was tiny, but not like a fetus at all, just like a tiny perfect baby. He had arms and legs and fingers and toes. At that moment I didn't know how anyone could not believe in God or believe in abortion because there at 13 weeks was my tiny perfect baby. I wanted to touch him and I wanted to take his picture but all I could do was cry. I looked over at Kevin and he was covering his eyes and sobbing. Then they took him away to perform pathology reports and to be picked up by the funeral home the next day. I got dressed and we were discharged home with a follow up with the OB the next day to ensure I had passed all the tissue. I don't remember much about that night except for sheer exhaustion and sleeping on a chucks pad because I was afraid I would bleed through my pants.

Kevin and I both took the rest of the week off work. The next morning when we woke up Kevin took care of calling the funeral home to arrange picking up the baby. At some point, Kevin also removed all evidence of the baby from view. He removed the ultrasound pictures from the fridge, erased the announcement from the chalkboard, moved that lion sleeper into the baby's room and closed the door to the baby room. I don't know if this helped or hurt. I wanted to remember him, but Kevin needed a fresh start. The hospital had actually called the night before so they were prepared. We made an appointment to go in that afternoon following my doctor's appointment. We went to the OB where they did an ultrasound to insure I had passed all the tissue. The ultrasound room was so oddly different than it had been just two days before. Kevin pumping his fist in the air, listening to a heartbeat…now just silence and sadness, the doctor determined that everything looked fine. We ate Fazoli's in the truck that day, then headed to the funeral home.

In the funeral home we chose, they have a sitting area in the back where people sit to make arrangements. I had sat in those chairs twice before, once as a sister and once as a daughter and that day I sat in them as a mother, I guess, to be honest, this put us in an odd situation…what exactly were we? We weren't parents, but we were something or we wouldn't be there. We discussed the burial of the baby, they offered all the traditional things—service, obituary, etc. but we just wanted to bury him. It really was an awkward place…not a human to most of the world but such a big piece of us. We opted to bury him on top of my dad, turns out that even for a coffin the size of a shoebox you have to pay the standard grave digger fee of $300. We would bury him the next day, in a simple service, me, Kevin and our preacher. It rained that day…I think it has rained every time I have buried an important man in my life. We brought the coffin my Grandpa made to the funeral home and Kevin put the knife I had given him for Father's Day in the bottom. There we stood in the rain with nothing much to say, except that God was in control. We went home where my mom had cooked lunch…that was it he was gone.

Facebook post-June 29, 2017: *"As some of you know, and some of you don't Kevin and I are no longer pregnant. Last night we miscarried our baby boy. After seeing our perfect little baby with his arms and legs and hands and feet, I can't imagine how anyone could believe in abortion or not believe in God. Words can't express our heartbreak or sadness. There are so many things we don't know or understand, but there are some things we know for sure. We know God is still God and he is still in control and even if he doesn't move mountains we want moved or part waters we want to walk through, we know it is well with our souls. And this…this is the best part, I know FOR SURE that when my precious baby boy opened his eyes for the first time he saw Jesus and his Grandpa (Nelson Adams) and it doesn't get much better than that for him, and one day…oh one day I will hold him in my arms. Thank you all for your kind words, thoughts and prayers, it truly takes a village of believers to live in this world."*

WE ARE PUBLIC NOW—2nd INFERTILITY LESSON LEARNED

This is when we learned the second major lesson from infertility. Sometimes God doesn't move mountains or part waters, but he is still in control and he is still God. Up to this point to be honest I haven't talked a lot about God. Of course, we were praying for our baby and for success every time, but I wasn't letting this teach me anything, I wasn't learning and I wasn't growing. For the most part, until we lost our son not a lot of people knew what we were doing, our families knew and very few close friends…but now, now all of Facebook and whoever had been told from people seeing it on Facebook knew what we were working towards and knew we were drastically failing. Being public changes things because now people are watching, wondering what you are going to do next and how you are going to handle it. Our preacher says a lot that sometimes you are the only Bible people read…how were we going to handle this and what were we going to learn from it. I told Kevin many, many times throughout this process that I wish we would hurry up and learn whatever it is God wanted us to learn so we could move on, but alas, it doesn't work that way. Sometimes you have to go through whatever your circumstances are to get to the end outcome. So to speak "You have to go through your go through to get to the end."

I call this time in our life the time when we drowned our sorrows in material things. Kevin hates when I call it that because it's not like we wasted tons of money and truthfully I did this more than him, but I did it. If I went somewhere and saw a purse or shirt or shoes or whatever and felt like I wanted it, I convinced myself I deserved it. Look what I had gone through, look at my bad luck, look at my sadness, I deserved whatever I wanted and I suppose at the moment I felt some good control over wanting something and being able to get it because the one thing I really wanted I was not able to get.

I don't remember the exact date but it was a week or two after we lost the baby that his pathology report came back. Kevin got it from medical records and brought it home. I will never ever forget that night. I made him promise not to read it without me and he obliged. As soon as he got home that night I wanted to see it. I read it right there in the driveway and I remember breaking down. I had only ever "broke down" one other time in my life (the night my brother died), but I lost it right there in the driveway. The pathology report was not exactly what I had expected. There were no "medical results," no blood or tissue just observations. Anatomy was normal, it was, in fact, a boy, and there were measurements to indicate all seemed typical no obvious signs of chromosomal abnormalities or sickness for all intents and purposes the baby was typical and the cause of the loss was not related to the baby and that's when it hit me. That meant the baby was fine and my stupid body couldn't keep him inside. I remember sobbing, you know the body-shaking, breath-losing, all-out sobbing on Kevin's shoulder before he even got out of his truck. I felt like my body had failed me like I was the ultimate failure of a woman, the baby was fine and my body just didn't do what it was supposed to do. I don't remember exactly what Kevin said but he comforted me and that's all that matters.

TURNING POINT—*Proverbs 3: 5-6: "Trust in the Lord with all your heart and lean not on your own understanding, in all your ways submit to him, and he will make your paths straight."*

At some point in the couple of weeks that followed I turned a corner, I adopted a new mindset. I decided that grief, mourning, sadness—those were all OK and those would always be a part of my life but I couldn't get stuck there.

Facebook post-July 13, 2017: *I posted an article that day titled "The Day God Gave Me More Than I Could Handle" and wrote this about it: "This!! 1000 times this!!! I promise I have been given more than I could ever handle on my own. The only reason I can get up every morning and put one foot in front of the other is that I believe God is there too, and I believe a miracle is coming!!!"*

"Jesus answered and said to him, "What I am doing you do not understand now, but you will understand later." –John 13:7."

KEEP YOUR HOPE, FIGHT FOR JOY AND BUY THE DIAPERS

That's when I adopted my mantra "Fight for Joy." I started buying diapers and clothes every time I went to the store. The door to the baby's room got opened again and the lion sleeper returned to my dresser knob where it would then hang until a baby wore it. I started filling that room that Kevin had shut the door on a month earlier, with diapers and clothes for a baby we did not have. "They" say that hope deferreth make the heart sick and that is so true. That's where I had been in the past month heart sick. One of Kevin's coworkers sent us a sympathy card following the loss and it had this verse in it: *"The Lord is close to the brokenhearted and saves those who are crushed in spirit." –Psalm 34: 18.* I lost it when I read that too because that is exactly what I was! Crushed in spirit, I had never heard it put exactly that way, you know there is sad and there is grieving, but CRUSHED in spirit that was me and it said that he was near to me and would save me.

Facebook post-July 15, 2017: *I posted a link to the song "Old Church Choir" By: Zach Williams and wrote this: "This song is my current favorite...listen to it! Several years ago I worked with a very wise physical therapist who told me this same message...we would often repeat it to each other. I have repeated this to myself many many times in the last couple of weeks. I have fought so hard to keep my joy (And y'all, it has been a Fight!), but I AM GOING TO KEEP IT! The Bible says hope deferreth make the heart sick, and I can attest to that! You must, I repeat must keep your hope. I am keeping a tight grip on my home...my hope for happiness, my hope for a baby...my* *miracle IS coming! And until then Ain't NOTHING gonna steal my JOY!!!! "Though he slay me, yet will I trust in him." –Job 13: 15.*

At some point, we returned to Dr. Griffin who told us we needed to take a short break following what they called a 13-week miss. He said that he would be willing to attempt again in an August cycle; however, wanted to repeat a couple of tests first just to be sure that everything still looked good. So that is what we planned.

Facebook post-July 20, 2017: *I posted a picture of that lion sleeper we had purchased so long ago (I guess I decided if we were going public, we were going all out) and wrote this: "To some of you this may be a onesie...to me, this is FAITH in a tangible form. In November of 2015, Kevin and I purchased this to start the process of preparing for a baby. A baby we had already been trying to get for almost a whole year. This is just the beginning folks...yes we have a half-done nursery, yes we have almost enough diapers to last the first year of our baby's life...no we don't have a baby...no we are not pregnant... BUT we will be one day! Faith is hard...I repeat hard! Our story is exposed, a story we kept hidden from most people for 2 years, but if it's going to be out there... then let it be for God's glory. Is my faith strong every day...nope, is my faith strong most days...nope, but am I still clinging to the tiniest bit of it... YES, and NEWSFLASH...that tiny tiny bit can move mountains!!! One day when we bring a baby home wearing this onesie I want you all to remember this, that onesie is as old as a toddler...whatever it is you need faith for tonight, maybe it's a baby like me or maybe it's a new job, or enough money to buy a house, or faith to save a family member....whatever it is cling to it with all you have left in you, because faith is what can make a blind man see, raise Lazarus from the dead, give me a baby, and answer your most fervent prayers."*

July 27, 2017: *I posted a link to the song Speechless by Steven Curtis Chapman and wrote this: "So…I am not, I repeat am not a singer, anyone in my family will second that, but I love to sing…in my car, and I am in my car a lot!!! So many songs with such great messages… this is an oldie but a goodie. Listening to it today and one particular line caught my attention. In the second verse, he says "to think, you still celebrate over JUST ONE who was lost." I REALLY started thinking about that. Sometimes we think what we want to do or say needs to reach hundreds or thousands to matter, but that's not the case…just 1…we need to reach just one and God celebrates just as big. This made me think of a couple things, what if I reach just one with a message, or reach just one with kindness, or just one with love…guess what?!?!?! That's as important as reaching 100. Also…I am that 1…God celebrated that big over just me…over just you and if just 1 matters that much…he ain't leaving me now. And I'm going to keep on keeping on because maybe today or maybe tomorrow or maybe next week my message or your message, or our love reaches just 1!!!! #justone #iveneverdonethehashtagthing"*

At this point, I started to immerse myself in positive things. I knew that I had to immerse myself in the word, in positivity and in joy if I was going to make it through this and keep any kind of hope and joy. When we started this journey years ago I wrote two Bible verses on a sticky note and stuck them to the refrigerator right by where you open the door so that I would see them every time I got in it. They were: "So keep up your courage, men, for I have faith in God that it will happen just as he told me."—Acts 27:25 and "Blessed is she who has believed that the Lord would fulfill his promises to her!"—Luke 1:45 and in fact they still hang on that same sticky note in the same spot to this day, but I decided that wasn't enough. I decided to start writing things on my bathroom mirror. At the end of July that year, my mirror had these three things written on it: "Pursue God more than you pursue a baby!"; "Though he slay me, yet will I trust in him…" –Job 13:15; and, "May he give you the desire of your heart and make all your plans succeed." –Psalm 20:4

Facebook post-July 29, 2017: *I posted a picture of that bathroom mirror and wrote this: "Have you ever heard the saying fake it till you make it? (I learned that saying in OT school, which should only slightly alarm you…haha). Sometimes what my head knows to be true my heart struggles to believe…and in those moments I MUST surround myself with things that help me fake it till I make it… or know it until I have the faith to believe it. This is my bathroom mirror. Over the last year, it has had a variety of sayings and verses on it…every day when I get out of the shower, and when I'm getting ready I am constantly putting these thoughts in my head. You must surround yourself with positive thoughts and positive people What you put in your head and heart is what is going to make you or break you. Find something that motivates you and fake it till you make it!!* **#dailymotivation #psalm20:4 #job13:15"**

Shortly after I made the above post a patient I had been working with asked to be my friend on Facebook. She had been my patient for a while and I would say we bonded. In fact, I was supposed to treat her the day after my miscarriage and she was canceled, when I came back to work she was so concerned about what was wrong but I just brushed it off, so to think if I accepted her friend request I would be "outed" yet again. I really struggled with it, but I accepted her request. The very next time I saw her the very first thing she did was hug me, she hugged me for a good minute or two, looked me right in the eye and nodded, as if to say…we don't have to talk about it, but I know and I am so so sorry. She was really my most favorite patient of all time, we would keep in touch even after she was discharged and even after I moved on from that job. She would actually come to my baby shower to celebrate with me. I will never forget that moment right there in the hallway of the waiting room, where we made a connection in my grief, a connection that didn't require any words…another lesson was learned right here a lesson to me to not be afraid to be "outed" because people care and they are rooting for me too.

HERE WE GO AGAIN...OR MAYBE NOT

August was here!! The month the doctor said we could try again. Everyone's infertility situation is different and some people have a chance even if it is small of conceiving outside the fertility clinic, Kevin and I, however, did not. If we were not actively in an IVF cycle we were NOT going to get pregnant. So when we were in the waiting I felt like we weren't doing anything and when we started a cycle, it was almost as though I got a sort of high from it. It is difficult to explain but there was an emotion that came with starting the meds that could not be replicated by anything else.

Facebook post-August 4, 2017: *I posted an article called: Emily lays down for ultrasound—but when tech goes quiet she knows something's terribly wrong—and wrote this: "This is truth! But there are other things they don't tell you. They don't tell you that this could happen again, and again and again. They don't tell you that during those weeks when your body is "cleaning out" and you think you can never do this again, that you can and you will. They don't tell you that when you miscarry it can feel like labor, they don't tell you that the "fetus" that isn't old enough to be considered life, will still look exactly like a baby. But they also don't tell you that you and your husband will grow closer with each tragedy, they don't tell you that God will become more real every time, they don't tell you that your faith will both be tested to its greatest bounds and at the same time grow beyond your wildest imagination. They don't tell you, you will be stronger for having made it through this with your joy still intact.*

Tragedy (of any kind, not just a miscarriage) is a test of faith…but whatever your tragedy is you are stronger for having conquered it… keep the faith, find the joy even in tragedy and sorrow…enjoy life, live till you die and pursue your biggest dreams!!!"

Facebook post-August 7, 2017: *I posted a picture of magic lilies in our yard and wrote this: "I love these! They are one of my most favorite flowers. We bought our house in June, imagine my joy when these bloomed in our yard in August, one of my most favorite features. Just as their name implies they are "magic." They are nowhere to be seen and then bam one day there they are and today I noticed them everywhere!! Just like these flowers folks our circumstances can change in an instant. Just like that life can be better or worse. These flowers are a great reminder to find the joy in where you are now. No, my life isn't going as I planned (not by the longest shot you can imagine), but it could be 1000X worse. There is joy everywhere. Joy in these flowers popping out today, joy that my husband and I are healthy, joy that we both have good jobs, joy in my family and friends, joy that the battle we are fighting is one we chose to fight, not one that was forced on us. Hope deferreth make the heart sick…I cling to my hope because tomorrow, or next week or next month my circumstances could be worlds different and I don't want to miss what's in store for me or miss the joy between now and then. So enjoy these flowers for the next week or two, because then they will be gone. Let them remind you that where you are now you don't have to stay!* **#magiclilies #findyourjoyandkeepyourhope***"*

Dr. Griffin had two requirements before we could proceed with another transfer. He wanted to redo a test that would allow him to get a good view of the inside of my uterus to ensure nothing in there could have caused the miscarriage and he wanted us to meet with a perinatologist which is a high-risk OB to insure that this doctor didn't recommend anything any different.

First came the appointment with the perinatologist. Both Kevin and I went, it was a lengthy visit that consisted of long histories of our families and our medical histories, we then met with a genetic counselor and then the doctor. Ultimately he had a few labs he wanted to run to double-check a couple of things (on a side note our insurance would later deem these labs not necessary and we would fight for over a year to get them paid for—which is ridiculous!) ultimately the tests came back normal but if they had been atypical it could have saved our future children. So this step done, onto the test…

This test involved a vaginal ultrasound and injecting saline into my uterus—thankfully it was not the same as the HSG—which was my very first question. This test was relatively painless, but while the test was going on I could tell something was wrong… this is the true test of how you tell if something is good or bad at the fertility clinic. If it is good news the doctor will just tell you during the test, or after you sit up, if it is bad news he will tell you to get your pants on and meet him in his office—I have experienced both multiple times. That day he had me get dressed and come to his office so I knew something was wrong. He told me that something showed up in my uterus and they needed to do surgery to investigate what it was before proceeding with a transfer. Here we go…it never ever goes as it should with IVF, if you plan on doing a round a certain month you might as well assume it will get postponed by at least two.

We scheduled the surgery and went in for it. It's odd to say but we had a pretty good day the day of the surgery. The surgery was scheduled for a little later in the day so we slept in and leisurely headed to Evansville, it was a nice day just Kevin and me. The surgery discovered that there was a piece of the placenta still in my uterus from the miscarriage. Dr. Griffin removed it and said it was good he did that test and found it. He also said that while he was in there he did some kind of uterus scratching thing that could possibly increase our chances of the next round working. He said the statistics weren't great for it that's why he doesn't do it all the time, but since he was already in there he might as well. The recovery from the surgery was easy, painless. We stopped and ate out on the way home. By the time everything was said and done we had missed the cutoff for August so the plan would be to proceed with a transfer in September…hurry up and wait some more.

Facebook post-August 11, 2017: *I posted a link to the song Roots by Unspoken and wrote this: "This song was written about ME!! (OK maybe not really, but that sounds pretty empowering to say). I love to belt this song out in the car. There is so so much truth here. Yes, I have been through a "drought," yes I have "withered in the snow" and been "bent by the winds"…BUT still, I haven't broke! How powerful is that statement but still I haven't broke!!! I'm saying it one more time because I like it…STILL, I HAVE NOT BROKE! And why…why am I still standing? Because I have firm, good roots. I have roots in Jesus Christ! And I am oh so so thankful for those roots. This last year and a half would have surely broken me if I didn't have those roots. I am so thankful for parents like Nelson and Christina Adams who raised me up with those roots, who took me to church, who taught me to pray and trust God even in the bad times (and goodness knows they had their bad times, to teach that in). I am so thankful for strong church families I grew up in like the First Baptist Church in Sesser and for the generations of good people there like Delbert Brown, Dean Webb and George Spotanski, men I used to love to hear pray…*

in these times of sorrow, I am so thankful for my roots that help me stay firmly planted in my hope and joy! Parents...make sure you're giving your kids good roots!!!"

August 18, 2017: *I posted the link to the song Broken Things by Matthew West and wrote this: "I'm back...listen to this one!! But guess what folks that #hope #joy I've been talking about...they've been gone this week, and I'm just being real. As much as I try to cling to them, sometimes they get stolen...but just for a little while. It's been a tough week, oh in the scheme of things it wasn't that bad (trust me I've had much, much worse), but...just being teal...this week was sucky, both because I had some yuck stuff happen, but also because I didn't handle all the yuck stuff with the grace I should have, sometimes #life steals your #joy! But...oh there's that BUT, this sone reminds me He uses the broken things (thank goodness!) It's that verse...the beggars and the prodigals, the humble and the weak... give me hope for sinners like me. Even when this life gets us down (because it will) that's when we fight with everything we've got for out #hope and #joy! So this weekend I'm appreciating my husband, who would do whatever he could to take my pain away, I'm spending some time with my mom who is my best friend and I'm gonna get close to Jesus! Next week I'm keeping my #hope and #joy!!!"*

Facebook post-August 18, 2017: *"God is within her, she will NOT fall. —Psalm 46:5"*

Facebook post-August 20, 2017: *I posted a Facebook memory from the year before of an article titled The Day God Gave Me More Than I Could Handle and wrote this: "A year later and this remains truer than ever!! There ain't nothing gonna steal my Joy!!! I fight for it every day!!"*

MAKING CHANGES TO
GET A BABY

⌒‿⌒

In the middle of August, I applied for a job. It was on a whim and super unplanned. A friend I went to undergrad school with notified me of a job opening in a school, I always wanted to work in a school and who can beat the schedule? But I knew it would be a large pay cut. In fact, the day before the interview I was going to call and cancel it but my husband talked me into going ahead and going. The interview went great and I was offered the job. I spent the next two days struggling hard over a decision. I wanted this job A LOT, but I also knew the pay cut would be HARD!! I crunched the numbers over and over but I just couldn't make them work. I ultimately turned the job offer down.

Facebook post-August 28, 2017: *I posted a link to the song "Eye of the Storm" by Ryan Stevenson and wrote this: "Another good one! There are several parts of this song that really stick out to me "when a sickness steals my child away, and there's nothing I can do"...now that hits home...and "I find my peace in Jesus name'... now that is a good one!!! There are so many days when life gets us down and the only place there is peace is in Jesus' name! I tell people I walk a VERY fine line between happy and sad...joyful and bitter, and most days I pull myself over to the happy and joyful side, but truth be told it doesn't take much to push me over that line and I can become sad and bitter in an instant!! But it's in those times I remember in the eye of the storm...he remains in control!! There are so many truths to this song, I am so thankful he guards my soul, my battle is deep (as is everyone else's) and the devil gets a hold of a lot of my stuff. My fam-*

ily, my joy, my job, my hope…but I always know Jesus is guarding my soul!! And that is the most important, I always know it is well with my soul. This song reminds me of the story in Matthew where Jesus falls asleep on the boat during the storm, but the disciples panic. That's me!!!! I'm the panicky disciple!!! When the storm is raging I panic, but there's no need!! Jesus has it all under control!! When the devil gets ahold of your battle, whatever it is, know that Jesus is there in the eye of the storm! #mypeaceinJesusname #bebetternotbitter #fightingdailyforhopeandjoy

Sometimes God has an interesting way of making sure we follow his plans. Two weeks after I turned down that job offer, I lost my job. The company I worked for was no longer going to be providing therapy in nursing homes and therefore didn't need as many employees. About 20 or more people lost their job the same day I did, including my two very best friends. I remember going into panic mode. I actually saw it coming if I'm being honest, but when it actually happened I panicked. I needed a job, we needed my income and I needed health insurance with no lapse if IVF was still in my future. Here I was expecting an IVF transfer in about two weeks and my world was crashing down.

Facebook post-September 1, 2017: *I posted a picture of my dad and wrote this: "Missing this guy something fierce tonight!! I'll tell you what, if you want to stir the devil up just tell him you're fighting for hope and joy…he will kick into overdrive! I'm claiming it now… there are two things I'm fighting for 1) A baby and 2) MY JOY! And I'm in the fight of my life for both, but I'm getting them and ain't NOTHING stealing them. This guy would have had some words of wisdom today…if only I knew what they were. Hanging onto this verse tonight "For I know the plans I have for you declares the Lord, plans to prosper and not to harm, plans for a HOPE and a future." —Jeremiah 29:11" #fightingforJoy*

September 2, 2017: *I posted a link to Facebook that said: "staying happy is a MUST. Praying is a MUST. Ignoring negativity is a MUST. Staying focus is a MUST. Remaining humble and grateful is a MUST" and wrote this: Yes! This!! 100X this!!*

I did call back about the job I had interviewed for and it was still available, I also interviewed for 3 other jobs and was offered them all…but now I had a hard decision to make.

Kevin and I had many conversations about the job offers. He wanted me to take the job that was offered in the school. After all, he was the one who initially wanted me to go to that interview. He wanted me to have that schedule and to be able to be off on holidays and in the summer with our future child, and while I appreciated all of that it would be a major financial change. I am a numbers cruncher and I struggled to make them crunch. But if I'm being honest part of my hesitation was the part about having that schedule to be home with our child. Of course, what mom wouldn't want that but in the back of my mind, I just kept thinking what if there is never a child to be home with?? In fact, I remember saying these exact words to Kevin "what if I am home summer after summer with no child?" This job would be a major sacrifice on both our parts financially. It was a big step.

Ultimately I took the school job, stepped out in faith. If what I was fighting for was Joy and a baby both of things would be easier to get with this job. If I truly believed God was going to give me what I wanted then I needed to start acting like it. So I accepted the job and would finish out the month of September in my current job, which meant I had time to squeeze one last IVF transfer in on this insurance and under the max out of pocket payment that had already been made.

In IVF, things never go as planned

Following the procedure in August we were all a go for the cycle in September, I was going to squeeze the transfer in before the change in insurance and all was great. They have you come in for baseline lab work right before all the meds start up. My mom took me to that appointment at the beginning of September. We went to get lab work done and then we were going to go fall flower shopping, you know pumpkins and mums, it was going to be a good day, a day full of joy.

It's odd the things that stick out in your memory after the journey is over, but this day is one that for some reason sticks in my head, I remember it was raining and I remember the raincoat I had on. I remember the back road we were on, on our way to the nursery for mums when the phone rang. I remember which nurse it was that called that day, Colleen and I remember what she told me. I wouldn't be able to proceed with the September cycle because it appeared I had just ovulated on my own, I would need to wait for my period and then sync up with their October cycle. I barely held it together on the phone and then just like it was yesterday I can remember losing it right there in the car. I just started bawling. This cycle was supposed to be perfect, the last one before my insurance changed, I would have been due in the summer while I was off from my new job and now the one thing my body seemed to never be able to do which was part of the reason for IVF in the first place, it had just done on its own exactly when it wasn't supposed to do it. My body was letting me down yet again!! I remember we pulled into the nursery and I refused to get out of the car. I couldn't pull myself together and besides, at that moment I didn't feel much like getting a pumpkin or a mum—my mom got me one anyway, but that day, I did not win the fight for joy.

Facebook post-September 13, 2017: *I posted a link to the song "The Comeback" by Danny Gokey and wrote this: "Stay tuned...I will have a comeback. I'm not sure when, because believe me God has made it extremely evident to me that the timing is not my choice...but I WILL have a comeback, and it will be BIG!!! The last couple of weeks have been WOW!!! That's really the only way to describe them...and they have not all ended how I would have wished...but that's ok because I don't write the story...he does, so just be ready because I'm not sure when, but MY miracle IS coming (and so is yours)!!!!*

The next few weeks there wasn't much to do on the IVF front except wait for my period (Oh yay!—insert eye roll) and focus on my job change. This job change was going to be huge, it was a totally different job than I had been doing, but also I was going to leave my two best friends. The two girls who had been with me through my whole journey, who knew things I wouldn't tell anyone else, the two girls who believed wholeheartedly as much as I did that I would have a baby one day. When I came back to work following my ectopic pregnancy I had a box waiting of comfort items, when I told them I had a miscarriage at 13 weeks, I was immediately offered meals, they listened about every appointment, every excitement and every letdown. IVF is not exactly a topic you broach with new coworkers for the fun of it. I was leaving my cushion so to speak.

Facebook post-September 22, 2017: *"Bear with me folks it's about to get cheesy and sappy up in here!!! These girls right here they are my ride or die (that's what people say right??), my BFFs (now I feel like I'm 12), for real they are what keeps me sane sometimes. Today was the last day the package deal, will be together at work! These girls have been there for me like you wouldn't imagine. They have made me goodie boxes, offered to bring me food, stood in funeral* lines, and loved me through it all the last couple of years. We have laughed together, cried together, complained together and adulted together (because sometimes it takes us all to make adult decisions). God knew what he was doing when he put us all together. I'm gonna miss you girls like no other!!!"

Facebook post-September 22, 2017: *"This is a long one folks…I struggle sometimes about what to post and what not to post, I don't want to cross the line and become an oversharer but I also feel like I want my story to be for something and it won't be if I keep it quiet, and a very dear friend of mine offered some encouragement this morning to keep it up, so here goes. A couple weeks ago I was offered my dream job, and I know that's super cliché but for real my DREAM job and I turned it down for monetary and insurance reasons (I feel I must mention at this point my husband encouraged me to take this job in the first place, in fact, he's the only reason I went to the interview and it has become apparent he was right the whole time!)…flash forward 2 weeks and the company I work for was forced to lay off 20 employees (myself included)…of course, my gut reaction was sheer panic… hello, I need a job, a paycheck and insurance!!!!! I won't bore you with the details, but this job and others were offered to me and I am so so thankful for these options and choices!!! This is where the "lesson" and God part came in. (Hang in there, I know it's long but I'm going somewhere) Remember the reasons I didn't take this job, those are still there…and some of the other jobs would have solved those problems…but it was time to walk the talk I've been talking for months!! The walking part is so so so hard!!! I am fighting for JOY and a BABY and both of those things will be easier to fight for at my new job, but for a few days, my mind wanted to fight for money and security and material things… that is not I repeat NOT what I am fighting for. I am so happy and thankful this job was still an option, I know it is 100% a God thing that it was "forced" into this job…now the last* *couple of weeks since accepting this job the devil has been in overdrive trying to convince me I needed those other jobs with more money and more security but I must remind myself daily I am fighting for JOY and a BABY, not money!!! I am so thankful for my time at Joyner therapy because it brought me 2 of the best friends a girl could as for, I met so many wonderful patients including my most favorite shoulder patient ever (you know who you are), and it served its purpose for the time, but better things lie ahead than what I leave behind!! So here's to good things to come (including snow days, Christmas break and summer vacation) at Kaskaskia Special Ed district!! Whatever you are fighting for know God is fighting right beside you!!! Just be ready to walk it out in faith!!!! #fightingforjoyandababy"*

Facebook post-October 3, 2017: *"Marriage is defined as the legally or formally recognized union of two people as partners in a personal relationship...but it is oh so so so much more than that. I never would have imagined what the last 3 years would hold. Kevin and I often joke that our worse came before our better and sometimes I believe that, but there is no one else I'd rather do life with than this good ball. Young people listen up...marriage is not rainbows and unicorns, marriage is not endless date nights, marriage is not cuddling every night...marriage is fighting and hoping you make up before you go to sleep, marriage is learning to give nightly shots to your wife when needles make you want to faint, marriage is loving each other when your world is crumbling. Marriage is sacred and marriage is beautiful, it is hard...but it is so worth it!! Kevin and I have made a house and home together, we have cried, prayed and laughed together and we have buried a child together...this is life and it's not grand and fancy, but it's ours!! I am so thankful God saved Kevin for me! He is my rock, he is my friend and he is part of my Joy!!! Happy Anniversary Kevin Stubblefield!"*

NEW JOB CHANGES
THE WHOLE PROCESS

I started my new job at the very end of September and was set-
tling in well, but it was time to start the October cycle before
I knew it. No one at my new job knew I was doing IVF which
complicated it slightly and my new job while it had a great schedule it wasn't as flexible as my old job, so instead of just moving
things around a little and working late or an extra day I had to
take time off for my appointments. Juggling the new job and the
appointments for this cycle proved that doing IVF with this job
was going to be harder.

Kevin and I had agreed that this would be the last IVF cycle but
it was always in the back of my mind that I would do this until
I had a baby. Dr. Griffin had told us he would not do more than
3 cycles for people if they had not conceived but he didn't count
our first cycle so in my head I knew I had one left. So while I
know Kevin was banking on no more cycles I was always thinking about more, but this October cycle showed me that we could
never do a full cycle again until the summer for sure.

Facebook post-October 12, 2017: *I posted a link to the song
"Your Love Defends Me" by Matt Maher and wrote this: "Another
good one!!! The end of the second verse is my favorite!! "Although the
battle, it rages on, the war already won, I know the war is already
won!!!" I belt this part out every time!! This is what I keep reminding
myself of, sometimes the battle is LONG and hard, but in the end,
the war is already won! This can apply to so so many things. My war*

for a baby, my war for joy, the war of life, your war for financial security, your war for salvation or your child's salvation, your war for sobriety, your war for happiness, your war for a spouse…you get the picture. Jesus has won the war!! The key is we must fight because the battle is raging on—in the end the war is won but only if we stay in the battle. We can't give up hope, we can't give up trying. Every day we must CHOOSE to do battle for the desires of our heart. We can't sit back and wait for them to appear we must battle and sometimes when that battle is deep and wide, when it looks like endless doctors' appointments or endless bills, or endless lonely nights we remember the war is already won!!!" ***#fightingforjoyandababy #battlehard #thankGodthewariswon***

Facebook post-October 15, 2017: *(October 15th is pregnancy and infant loss remembrance day)—"I remember this day last year, I had lost one baby to a miscarriage at 7 weeks and I thought about posting something, but at that time our story was still, for the most part, pretty private and lots of people have had miscarriages so I just let it go…but this year, I have lost 4 babies. That miscarriage, a bilateral ectopic pregnancy and the most recent miscarriage at 13 weeks, so much has changed, so much of our story has changed and so much of my mindset has changed. Today (really every day) I remember those babies. I think about what could have been my 7-month-old baby, or my 2-month-old twins, or the fact that I could be 6 months pregnant. I think about how I felt last year, and the fact that I didn't value that one miscarriage enough, that just because it happens to lots of people doesn't make it easier or "no big deal." I think about the impact on my life (and hopefully other people's lives) those 4 babies have had, I think about what those 4 babies have taught me…they have reminded me that life can change in an instant, they have taught me to fight for Joy—NO MATTER your circumstances and they have taught me to love deeper. If I could talk to those ba-*

bies I would tell them how sorry I am, that I had to lose so many of them before I understood, the importance of joy and love. Only one of those babies made a tangible entrance into my life and he is now buried surrounded by 2 of the most important men in my life. Today I remember those babies a little extra and know they aren't lost…they are where their soul belongs and I will hold them in my arms someday. Today I remind myself to keep my hope and to fight for my joy… today I am thankful for those 4 babies and the impact they have had on my life and my walk with Jesus." **#keepingmyhope #fightforjoy #rememberthemeveryday**

Facebook post-October 16, 2017: *I posted pictures of my dad and posted this: "Oh how I miss this old guy!!!! Tomorrow is his birthday…61, there's not much I wouldn't give or do to have a party with him tomorrow, but alas that is not a choice. He has gone on, he fought the fight, he finished the race and he kept the faith. I have thought so much about him these last couple of months, oh what advice he would have had in my recent job change, and oh the joy that must have been present when he held my baby in heaven. I do not know how heaven works, but I know the Bible says we will be known as were known and because of that, I have no doubt he has held my sweet boy. As some of you know and some of you don't my dad was not a healthy man in his last few years here, but he refused to go to the doctor (I know if you knew him, this is not a shock). One day when trying to convince him he needed to go I reminded him how hard Kevin and I were trying to have a baby and how much I wanted him to be here for that baby…he calmly and wholeheartedly told me he without a doubt would be…he is not here, but he is there with my baby and I think of that statement often and how much truth neither of us realized that statement held, he is there where I cannot be. My dad taught me so many lessons in life, he taught me a good work ethic, he taught me how to shoot a gun, he taught me to love Jesus and* *he taught me how to keep living even during tragedy. My dad fought very hard for his joy! It does my heart good to know he is no longer fighting, he is in glory, he is home where his soul belongs!! And one day I will join him there, but until then I'm going to live, I'm going to hope and I'm going to fight for joy!!! Happy birthday, Dad!!!!"*

October 25, 2017: *"A friend of mine (Jody Moore), posted a thought today and I LOVED it so much!!! I wanted to steal it for myself!!! Just because I have grief in me does NOT mean I am without happiness and joy!! She is on point with this...grief is there it will always be with us, whatever scars we have they are there forever...but that does not mean we can't also have happiness, hope and joy!! And some days that grief reaches DEEP and gets us...but we MUST not wallow in it...because that happiness and that joy they are still there and we must fight for them!!! Thank you so much for the reminder today Jody!!!"*

We proceeded with a transfer in October, at this point Dr. Griffin was only willing to transfer one embryo at a time which also frustrated me. I understood his reasoning, we had had so many odd issues that it was not smart to possibly create another issue by getting pregnant with multiples. So here we were towards the end of our embryos, they implant them in quality order, so to speak, these last two embryos were lower quality and now they would only implant one at a time. Transfer went as normal...commence pee on a stick marathon, except this time nothing happened. The second line never showed up. It had been a while since we did a cycle with no kind of hope.

By the time I had the blood test and they called with the results I was pretty prepared, I didn't even cry on the phone. (I know I've already said it before, but it's so odd how seemingly normal things stick out in our mind later). I remember like it was yesterday standing in the parking lot of my office talking to the nurse who told me I was not pregnant. I didn't even cry this time, and setting up when to start everything to transfer our last embryo in November...but that's the thing about marriage, it wasn't solely my decision when to complete the next transfer...

KEVIN HAD DIFFERENT PLANS

When Kevin and I got a chance to discuss the last embryo and when to transfer it, he told me he wanted to take a break. He was tired of seeing me sad month after month and did not want to spend the holiday season like that. He also felt like my body needed a break. I did NOT want to take a break. It is so hard to explain the high I got when completing an IVF cycle when I knew there was a chance I could get pregnant and the low I felt when I was doing nothing to further my chances. But in marriage exists great compromise. Ultimately we agreed to wait until January to transfer our last embryo. That would give us two months to enjoy the holidays, to relax, to enjoy each other and to focus on other things, to fight for our joy and to find it everywhere even in the small things.

Facebook post-October 29, 2017: *"We took a trip to the ark this weekend. What a sight to behold!! I oftentimes think I have great faith (though it wavers often and a lot), but after seeing something like this and really focusing on a man like Noah…I know my faith is weak. Can you imagine.. 1 man and his family the only ones believing in God, in the world…but he never doubted, it had never rained before…yet he never doubted. It took him possibly 50+ years to build the ark…and yet he never doubted. Can you imagine the ridicule and mocking…and yet he never doubted. When I think of the piddly things that make me doubt, I am ashamed. My new mantra while fighting for my joy, I'm going to have faith like Noah!!! #fightingforjoy #keepingmyhope #faith likeNoah"*

At the end of that trip to the ark, Kevin got sick. I won't go into a lot of details to save his dignity but it was TERRIBLE. We ended stopping at an ER somewhere in Kentucky on the way home and the three of us, him, me and my mom had never been so glad to actually get home that night. I don't do a lot for Kevin, I think sometimes people assume I do more than I do, but he is really independent, but in this sickness, he required A LOT!! When we got home and I got Kevin settled in our room my mom and I were sitting in the kitchen and I remember saying to her that maybe this is why we weren't able to have a child. That we really couldn't handle it, that God knew what he was doing and we didn't need a baby and it was at that moment that I truly started to question whether I would ever have a baby and whether I really could handle a baby. The questioning was short-lived though, that's the thing, doubt, sadness, etc. these things creep in on us sometimes but we have to shut them down. I was scared, the Bible says that God will give us the desires of our heart, but I was scared I would never get mine.

ADOPTION AGAIN...

Facebook post-November 6, 2017: *"There's not much to say that hasn't been said before. Tomorrow is this guy's birthday. He would have been 32...if only things had gone differently. I can't help but to sometimes think about what life would be like if he were still here—but there's really no need for that as we cannot change our situation. I would love to be partying tomorrow but it is not so. I will remember a little extra tomorrow, but instead of getting swallowed up by grief, I will use tomorrow as a reminder that life is short and we must live while the living is good. So while I may have to fight a little extra for my joy tomorrow, you better believe I'll still be fighting. Happy birthday, Bubby, until I see you again in paradise!!"*

Facebook post-November 9, 2017: *I posted a Facebook memory from 2014 "At ANY given moment, you have the power to say this is not how the story is going to END" and wrote this: "This memory popped up today. It is from 3 years ago...so so much has changed in that 3 years. The girl who wrote that quote had no idea what was coming and how true that statement would be, and I am grateful for that. Had I known 3 years ago the battles I would fight and the outcomes, I'll just be honest I may have chosen not to fight them and I would have missed so so much!! As raw and ugly as the battles have been I wouldn't trade them now, I am so much closer to God and closer to Kevin, I know just how important my joy is and I will hold those babies one day! Still today...I LOVE this!! My story is NOT, I repeat NOT going at all how I wanted it to go...but you know what...it is going exactly how God wanted it to go (and as rough as things can get, there is so much comfort in that statement* *right there). In the middle of my story, right now, things are not going like I want…but I know the ending (because the war is already won). That may mean that I don't get to the end like I thought I would—God may have a different route, but I am NOT giving up!! My story is NOT ending here! I must fight for the ending I want!! #valuewhatyouvesurvived #fightingforjoy #fightingforababy #fightingformyending"*

The time off gave me a lot of time to think about things, which can be dangerous! There's a song I like to listen to and it has a lyric that goes like this: "There's a reason the road is long, it takes some time to make your courage strong." That is beyond true. There are so many things I did not have the courage to do in the beginning of our journey that I needed to do now. The courage to try again, to keep believing, to buy diapers and to surrender to God's will. It really started to impress upon my heart that we were not doing EVERYTHING in our power to get a baby.

This is when we started talking about adoption again. The concerns I had last time were still there but I was feeling stronger about the possibility of doing this. I feel like God was asking us, were we really doing whatever it took to get our dream?? Were we really willing to stretch ourselves? Which as I type that seems odd, ummm multiple rounds of IVF stretched us financially, emotionally and physically but it was still my comfort zone. To have a baby that's what I wanted, but what was more important?? Having a baby? Or raising a child and having a family?

We interviewed with a different agency this time called Everlasting Adoptions, it was a similar situation to before, we underwent a phone interview and were selected, but had to send them a LARGE sum of money to proceed. This time we decided to go ahead. We had one embryo left, the worst quality of this cycle, all we had done before was fail we were pretty sure it wouldn't work and we had agreed we would be done, so this would be our next game plan. Part of it I'm sure was my constant need to be "doing something" that was working towards getting my baby, but also we made peace with the fact that we may never have a baby that was biologically ours.

Once we signed up with the agency the next step was to get a home study completed. Now by this time, I can't even begin to count the times or ways my hoohaa had been prodded and by how many people but that was minimally invasive next to a home study. They dove straight into rocky territory. We filled out what felt like mountains of paperwork and then began the first of 3 interviews. The social worker came to our home which was scary to evaluate its readiness for a child and to talk to us. Kevin showed her our baby closet full of clothes while she was here, she was not impressed, in fact, she told us it was better not to prepare ahead of time too much because you may get tired of looking at things being empty…first of all…may get tired of it, lady we are already tired of it and number 2, we are going to prepare until I hold that baby in my arms because failure is not an option!! We hit a couple of snags on the way but ultimately got her all the paperwork she required to proceed with interview number 2…which is where they interview you about your childhood then split you up and interview you about each other. My interview with her lasted approximately 5 minutes, then Kevin's lasted approximately 30…I guess that's what happens when you mix two social workers!

Facebook post-November 15, 2017: *I posted the link to the song Hard Love by Need To Breathe and wrote this: "This is another good one, it took me a while to get into it…but once I did…SO much* *truth in this song! I would change one lyric though..."what doesn't kill ya CAN make you stronger" I would add that can...whatever we go through in life CAN make us stronger or not...it can be for good or it can be for naught. Our outlook, how we handle the situation can make us or break us. In the beginning, when I started my journey 3 years ago, I was not letting what didn't kill me make me stronger, in fact, I'd say it was making me weaker, I was cowering behind it in secrecy...but now I am so so much stronger, I have learned so so much from it, I have fought!!! I also love the line that says "there's a reason that the road is long, it takes some time to make your courage strong" ...SO MUCH TRUTH!! There are things I have had to do, especially recently that I never would have been able to do in the beginning because my courage wasn't strong. I have heard the saying many times, you have to go through, your go through and this puts a new spin on it, the road has been long, but oh my courage has grown strong. And maybe, just maybe what God has in store for me...takes a little extra courage (because goodness knows, it's not what I thought was in store) and this long road has prepared me!! #gettingpreparedforGodsplan #fightingforjoy #fightingforababy*

We finished our paperwork for the adoption agency and our home study shortly before Christmas...we became live with the adoption agency. Technically speaking we could get a call any moment about the baby that was waiting for us. Cue my extremely enthusiastic naivety...I was sure that phone call was coming any day!!

CHANGING MY MINDSET

During the holiday season of 2017 I truly, truly had the mindset change that I believe had to happen from the beginning. When you are trying to get pregnant everyone tells you to not want it so bad and it will happen (which it must be noted, is stupid advice!), and I always thought but you don't understand the preparation that has to happen, the money that has to be spent to make this happen for us we will never do it and not want it and then I started to reevaluate my mindset.

I started to find the joy in the smaller things in life. I started to really evaluate myself and God's plan for me. The Bible verse about God giving you the desires of your heart had been my go-to for so long, but I realized I wasn't approaching that correctly. When my dad died I questioned that a lot because I knew that his heart's desire was to not suffer and not end up on any machines and had he lived that night he would have encountered both those things, but my heart's desire was for him to live and he did not, so how could God give everyone the desires of their heart?? That's when I had a lightbulb moment I was thinking too shallow. I always thought a baby was the desire of my heart but truthfully my true heart's desires were things like hope, joy and happiness. I decided that God's way was not my way and I started praying for his will in my life rather than a baby. This was a giant shift!! I started praying for what I WANTED but KNOWING that whatever happened GOOD things were coming for me. Throughout the holiday season of 2017 that was my exact prayer. LORD, I WANT this last embryo to work, I WANT to have a baby, but

Lord, I KNOW if those things do not happen whatever you have in store for me is even better than that, because GOOD things are coming for ME!!

Facebook post-November 22, 2017: *"Thankful list 2017—It is so easy to get drug down by life. This life is full of sorrow, but when we purposely shift our thoughts to our blessings life instantly improves! It is so interesting to me to look back on lists form years back and to see how my perspective has changed. So without further ado here is my every day of thankfulness list for 2017: I am thankful for/that—*

1) *Jesus came to give me life more abundant.*

2) *Jesus completed the plan when he died for my sins.*

3) *Because of these first 2 items, I will see my dad and brother again and hold my babies in my arms.*

4) *Kevin—even though we have our not so loving moments, there is no one I'd rather do this life with.*

5) *My mom! And that she has had such a good and positive year.*

6) *My dad, and though he is gone his influence is deep.*

7) *Kevin's family and that they have also become my family.*

8) *I have a warm place to sleep every night.*

9) *Mine and Kevin's health.*

10) *I have made it through this year with my joy intact!!*

11) *My new job opportunity!*

12) *I now work for a school system and we don't work weekends and believe fully in holiday breaks!*

13) *Even when life doesn't go as we planned, God is still in control.*

14) *Friends—old and new and old friends that have resurfaced to become new friends.*

15) *I have no idea what it's like to actually be hungry.*

16) *Memories and pictures that help us remember the past.*

17) *I live in a place where I still have freedom.*

18) *The men and women who have fought for that freedom.*

19) *My struggles and battles this year, for they have taught me so much.*

20) *I am not the same person I was when I started my battles.*

21) *My hope!*

22) *My happiness!*

23) *All the good things I know are in store for 2018!*

Here's to another trip around the sun and I already can't wait to see what makes next year's list! Happy Thanksgiving!!"

There's that naivety again, I truly truly believed 2018 would be a good year and would bring me a baby!

Facebook post-November 24, 2017: *"Well as tradition goes, black Friday kicks off the Christmas season in the Adams/Stubblefield homes, and if you know me at all you know I live for Christmas!! I LOVE the whole Christmas season, I have most of my presents bought by September and wrapped before October is over...but this year I have been struggling with the Christmas season coming. It was this time last year that we found out about our ectopic pregnancy, and the due date form our most recent loss is quickly approaching...this year was supposed to be oh so different, but then I stop and remind myself that CHRISTmas and this season has nothing to do with how many kids I have, instead it has everything to do with God and*

his promise to us for eternal life. When I think about what Christmas really means, and that because of Christmas we have Easter and because of those we have eternal life and hope and JOY!! I can't help but become so thankful that God sent his son as a baby o grow up and die for MY sins. So this Christmas season whether your life circumstances are exactly how you want them, or you wish you had one more stocking over the mantle, or you wish your family was speaking to each other or if you don't have the money for presents, just remember what the Christmas season really means and that "spirit" everyone talks about will come a little easier!! So here is to Christmas season kickoff and everything it means!! Merry Christmas!!
#havingChritmasspiritevenif #fightingforjoyandababy

IT'S NICE WHEN OTHER PEOPLE HAVE YOUR BACK

⁓ ‿ ⁓

When we started this whole journey we really told minimal people about our situation and struggle. Of course, our mothers and Kevin's sister knew some of what was going on as did my grandparents, beyond that maybe each of us told a good friend and our preacher knew, as things carried on and with several losses we became public and while people didn't know exactly what was happening people knew we were struggling.

On November 26, 2017, I got this message from my cousin's wife:

Jessica: "Good morning Mariah, so I just wanted to let you know you have been in my mind and heart a lot. I pray for you and Kevin all the time. Yes, I am sitting here in church sending this too. We had a baby dedication this morning and I was asked to sing Hannah Prayed by Jeff and Sheri Easter. I haven't been able to practice the song all weekend without crying. Well, I didn't get through it this morning either. I am thinking of you today and praying. We love you guys. What is next for you guys? Please feel free to tell me you don't want to talk about it. I want to pray specifically for whatever you guys are praying for.

Me: "Thank you so much for thinking of us! We do usually keep things pretty close to the vest, but we also aren't ones to turn down prayers. We have one frozen embryo left but have decided to postpone that transfer until after Christmas to get through the holidays without the hormone use and disappointment. So provided everything goes as planned (which we have come to learn basically it never does) we will transfer that embryo in the middle of January. For now, we have decided that will be our last attempt at IVF, we just can't continue to afford it and it is too difficult to take all the time off work (it may be something we pursue again down the road, but as of now we will be done). Because of that decision, and because we have decided it is less important to have a child than it is to be a family we have also signed up with an adoption agency. We are knee-deep in the home study paperwork, which frankly sucks!!! But that should be done by the end of the year, and technically speaking we could get a phone call at any time then for a baby. We have opted to only pursue infant adoption at this time, which means the baby will be ours from birth. We know that it is ALL in God's hands. We may end up with a baby both ways and we certainly wouldn't turn that down either. To be honest we have stopped praying specifically for things (I mean we, of course, would love the transfer to take and I often pray for the mother out there that is choosing life right now instead of abortion for what could be "our" baby) but rally right now we are just praying for A BABY. A healthy baby that is ours. No one else knows about these plans except the 3 people who have had to write reference letters for us and our moms. But we will take all the prayer we can get!! Thank you again so much for thinking of us."

Jessica: "We will definitely be in prayer. I am sure you have but have you considered a surrogacy? Just wondering if that was an option for y'all.

Me: "Thank you!!! We really haven't thought about that because it really wouldn't help the issue. A large part of the issue is

Kevin's disability once we get the eggs, I technically should be able to carry them just fine, the ectopic and the last miscarriage were absolute flukes according to multiple doctors. Warning.... long explanation and TMI ahead...(I proceeded to tell her our story)...I have made more trips to Evansville at the butt crack of dawn before work than I can count and I have had so many shots they don't even phase me anymore. I want a baby more than I've ever wanted anything in the world and I have come to realize I can't make it happen...God is the giver of life. I really don't know why I told you the whole story I guess I just needed to get it out and you seemed a little interested. Haha. We don't talk about it a lot because I'll likely cry if we do and we try not to dwell on it, but I don't mind answering questions...it is an interesting thing IVF and infertility and it needs more awareness. We could seek a sperm donor, but if the baby isn't going to be "ours" then it just seems adoption should be the way to go. Kevin could have adopted a long time ago, but it took me a long time to come to terms with it. I will always miss carrying my child, and breastfeeding them and trying to decide if they look more like me or Kevin, but raising a child and having a family is more important than all of that. When I say I fight for joy, I mean that...every day I fight, but I am WINNING!!! And I hope my story is helping someone else too. I'm sorry again for the long story! But thank you so so much for the prayers and the interest! Also, I listened to that song today after you sent that message. I had never heard it before. And I got to thinking how neat would it be for this message to go full circle and you to sing that someday at my baby dedication. So keep practicing, you will need to be ready. My miracle is coming!!"

JESSICA: "Oh my goodness, Mariah, you have been through so much. You can talk to me ANYTIME! I mean it. I so wish there was something I could do for you guys. I will continue to pray for you and Kevin's miracle. Love you guys."

ME: "Praying is ALL any of us can do. And knowing that other people want it for us as much as we want it means so so much! Love you guys too!"

JESSICA: "I want it for you SO bad. I am going to pray you can carry a baby also. Being a mother is an amazing job! So I will also pray for that too."

ME: "Thank you!!!!"

This message taught me that people cared and wanted to pray for us, they wanted our success. Oh, I always knew that, but it was nice to know someone wanted it for us just as bad as we wanted it.

TRUE CHRISTMAS JOY

Facebook post-December 1, 2017: *"This Christmas count-down has been around for as long as I can remember My brother and I used to fight about who got to put the ornament up for the day and we would rearrange them to make sure we got to put up our favorites...the soldier in day 22 was always his. This now hangs in my house, I insisted it move with me. I look so forward to this every year (I really do turn into a 7-year-old at Christmas time), and this morning when I got to hang up number 1 I was filled with JOY! You see this is the key to fighting for joy, you must find it in the smallest things. Look, truth be told I do not have joy, most days, in fact, I don't have joy right now but I am fighting (pardon my French) like hell for it right now. And this morning when I put that ornament up I was filled with childhood memories and true joy!!! I know that my life could be so much worse, in fact I know there are people right here in my community fighting for their life instead of joy, and I know how blessed I am that that is not me, but that does not mean the I (or you) am without struggle. Everyone fights their own battles. So even if overall right now I'm struggling...in that moment this morning, I had pure joy, and that's the key folks, you may not always HAVE joy, but you must always be FIGHTING for your joy...and in that don't miss the tiny things...for they could bring you Great JOY!! Happy first day of December!! **#fightingforjoyandababy #Christmasspiritevenif"***

Facebook post-December 5, 2017: *I posted a link to the song "A Strange Way to Save the World" by Rascal Flatts and wrote this: "It's Christmas! (And if you read my posts you already know how I feel* *about that!) so, of course, my songs are Christmasy!! The chorus of this song really hit me today.., "I'm not one to second guess what angels have to say, but this is such a strange way to save the world." Think about it for real…he sent a baby…born of a virgin to save the WHOLE world…. Everything about that sentence is strange, and yet it was perfect! What if…just what if God has a strange way for whatever it is you are wanting (again if you read my posts, you know what I want). What if the way you're going to get what you want or are fighting for is not the way you planned or thought or even wanted. Isn't it that much better to know you're getting it the way God wanted. I have had to rearrange my thinking. I have quit praying for specific things and just started praying for God's will…I am going to do everything in my power to get what I want and then pray for his will to be done and however, he accomplishes that…I know it will be great! So maybe the way you're going to get what you want is not anywhere near how you thought it would happen…who are we to second guess? After all, he sent a baby to save the world!!! #fightingforjoyandababy #Chritmassongshaveagreatmessagetoo"*

I hated Kevin's plan to wait those 3 months at the time, but I will always, always believe that was the BEST decision now. That Christmas season of waiting I found the true desires of my heart, I found joy, hope and happiness—even without a baby. I let other things go and I truly found JOY!! *"These things I have spoken to you, that my joy may be in you, and your joy may be full. –John 15:11"* I learned a very valuable lesson that holiday season that I carry with me still to this day, I learned that grief and joy can coexist, I'm going to say it one more time, GRIEF and JOY can COEXIST! I will always have grief, I have endured a lot of loss but I will also always have JOY because I have endured a lot of good things too.

Facebook post-December 23, 2017: *"It's almost Christmas!! And most of the time this time of year, I get caught up in the hustle and bustle of the season, but occasionally on a quiet evening, I can start sinking in my grief. Thinking about what could have been. Christmas of 2014, Kevin and I started talking about having a baby, and oh the excitement of thinking that the next Christmas we would have a child…3 years later and here we are on Christmas eve, even with no reason to build gingerbread houses or go get the Santa picture at the mall. When I think back to Christmas of 2015 and I think how I didn't savor it enough…how I didn't soak up enough his need to change out of his pajamas before we opened present (it annoyed the crap out of me that he wouldn't stay in his pajamas to open present on Christmas morning!), or how he would get in "eat mode" after his nap while we watched the 3rd or so round of A Christmas Story… Christmas will never be the same without my dad. But when I start to sink in my grief, instead of wallowing in it, I try to climb my way out I remember how blessed I am that I'm able to celebrate Christmas and that I have a new job that allows me to have the next week and half off! And I know that I need to soak up this quiet evening, because there is hope that next Christmas eve, eve I might be starting new kinds of traditions with my own child (here's to hoping 2018 is our year!!), and I can rest assured this quiet evening that my dad is spending Christmas with the man that is the reason for the season and I can't even begin to imagine what that celebration is like!! And then I look around at the quiet house with the lit Christmas tree and I am filled with JOY!! In the next few days, I know there will be times I will be overtaken by a wave of sadness thinking about what I'm missing…but I'm going to dip deep and fight for my joy…in the big and the little things. May your next few days be filled with both the hustle and bustle of the season abut also may they be filled with pure JOY!! Merry Christmas!"*

Shortly before Christmas, we became "active" with the adoption agency. We were home study approved and had a profile both paper form and online—we technically could be called for a baby at any time. I remember sitting on the couch typing the above post of Facebook then I checked my email and I had one from the adoption agency...there was an available baby! I don't remember all the exact circumstances but I remember they were rocky...mother had a history of drug use, possible special needs, I don't remember all the circumstances but I remember knowing this was not the baby for us and yet still wanting to jump at the chance. It was an odd feeling...turning down a baby so to speak. That's when I realized this process was going to be difficult...how many babies would we have to turn down to find our baby and how would we know they were supposed to be ours??

Between Christmas and New year's I began the oral meds for the IVF round we planned to do in January...our last embryo. I hated some of the meds, there were days I took 8 or 10 pills some of which had very undesirable side effects (the kind that renders you close to the toilet) and it became a chore each evening, but with this round and my new attitude I started a tradition, and I started thanking God for something with each pill, it ranged from something that happened that day, thankful for this opportunity, thankful for my health, or Kevin's, but always with the last pill I thanked him for the little embryo in the freezer. It's true what they say when I thought about all the things I had to be thankful for it was much easier to find JOY!

Facebook post-December 30, 2017: *"Warning: Long year-end post!! Last year on New Year's Eve I made a post about how bad 2016 was and how ready I was to kick it to the curb and knowing how* great 2017 was going to be. Now as 2017 is wrapping up (goodness how has it been a whole year?!?!?) I find myself reflecting on it. If I were to look at 2017 through the same eyes I was using at the end of 2016, I feel I could say all the same things about 2017 being as terrible as 2016...but I don't have the same eyes I did this time last year. In truth 2017 was not near as good as I was hoping it would be or thought it would be, the main things I wished to gain in 2017 did not happen and some things I never dreamed I would lose were lost in 2017, but just as I said last year, a year is but a blip on the radar screen of our life and during this small blip I have grown so so much! I did not get to bring home a healthy baby in 2017 but I did get to experience the joy of seeing a positive pregnancy test and seeing that heartbeat on the screen if only for a few short weeks. I may have lost my job in 2017 but I gained my dream job and have extremely enjoyed Christmas break!! My relationship with God has grown beyond measure in 2017 and I have learned that he has my best interest in his hands and while I think I know what I want and need he knows far far better! My relationship with Kevin has also grown beyond measure in 2017, as he continued to be my rock. I have watched my mom transform herself this year looking like a whole new woman and fighting for herself! And...folks for the big finish...2017 is ending and I have KEPT my joy!!! I haven't had it every day this year but ultimately I am ending 2017 with my joy still intact, (and pardon my French but I have fought like hell to end the year that way). On January 1st last year I wrote 3 goals on each bathroom mirror in our house, 1 for me, 1 for Kevin and 1 for a friend of ours...the only one that was met was the one for our friend but you know what that's ok...because we learned and gained things this year we didn't even realize we needed. So this year I am ready to kick 2017 to the curb also, but not because it was so awful, but because I have Hope that 2018 will be my year, my miracle is coming and there's no reason it can't be this year, and because I want to see what JOY 2018

will bring us!!! No new year's resolutions here I'm just going to keep fighting for my joy!!! Here's to 2018! "Forget the former things, do not dwell on the past. See I am doing a new thing!"— Isaiah 43: 18-19.
#keepingmyhope #fightingforjoyandababy"

Facebook post-January 1, 2018: *"Blessed is she who has believed that the Lord would fulfill His promises to her. –Luke 1:45"*

Facebook post-January 3, 2018: *I posted a link to the song "All My Hope" by Jeremy Crowder and wrote this: "I was not…I repeat Not ready for Christmas break to be over, but I did enjoy my car and radio time again today! I drive quite a bit for work and my time in the car is my me and Jesus time and I crank that radio and praise God! Today I heard this one (and trust me…it was cranked), it got me thinking. I am so glad my yesterday is gone (what an appropriate song for the new year) because my sins are forgiven like this song talks about but also because my past failures are gone!! It's no secret what I've been working for and through human eyes, I have failed miserably at that. In fact, some people would look at me and think what a fool…give up already move on (and for the record this applies to so so much more than my fight for a baby, in fact maybe people have said it to you about a fight for something else), but you know what, in Jesus, my failures are gone, they don't matter, it's like I have a clean slate!! Now if my hope was in modern medicine or science, it would be hopeless and I would be a fool…because so far they have gotten me nowhere (now don't get me wrong, I 100% believe science and medicine have a place—remember I am a medical professional after all, but I believe God uses them, they are nothing on their own) but ALL my hope is in Jesus and because of that even with a poor track record I have just as much hope as someone with a perfect record! And for that, I am so grateful! And because my hope is in Jesus I know he is always working on my behalf. He wants better for me than I could* *ever think or imagine, which made me think—I know how bad I want something, and when I don't get what I want when or how I thought I wanted it, imagine how much better whatever he has in store for me is going to be! Because as great as I thought things were going to be whatever he has coming is 100X better!! Thank God my yesterdays are gone and ALL my hope is in Jesus because I have good things coming!!"* **#keepingmyhopeinJesus #mymiracleiscoming #fightingforjoyandababy**

HERE WE GO FOR
THE LAST TIME

Message to Jessica: January 7, 2018

ME: *"So since you asked a while back what to specifically pray about, I'm going to share something with you. Friday we will have our final frozen embryo transferred. We have decided we will not pursue IVF anymore after this. I have had a true change of heart through the last few years. I want this just as much now if not more as when we started but I am to the point that I know if it doesn't work, it's because something better is coming. That has become my mantra of the last few weeks when I start to worry about it not working I repeat to myself that whatever he has in store is going to be great so if it's not this it just means something better is coming. With that being said I cannot express how bad I want this to work and God and I have had that conversation a lot the last couple of weeks too, that I am ok if it doesn't because I know he has good things for me, but I want this sooo bad. So I said all that to say this…if you would still like to, I would be honored if you would pray specifically that this transfer results in a healthy baby for us. We aren't telling anybody except our moms and you…but I know the power of prayer and if you're offering I'm certainly not going to turn it down. If you have any questions I don't mind answering them, that was a lot of info."*

Jessica: *"Of course I want to. I will pray what you want but also for His will to be done. You are His child and He wants the best for you. I feel very blessed to be able to pray for you and Kevin. Love you all."*

Me: *"Thank you so much! The next 2 and half weeks of waiting may be the hardest part of the whole thing!"*

Jessica: *"I will pray that goes fast also."*

Before we knew it the day was here. January 12, 2018, I remember the details of that day like it were yesterday, the day the last embryo would be implanted in me. I actually had the day off as a snow day—actually an ice day but that didn't stop us from making the trip to Evansville. Just like always, we stopped at a rest area to pee shortly before getting there then downed that water all 64 oz of it. When you go in for the transfer the first the nurses always asked as you were getting settled in the cubicle was how your bladder felt...FULL and if you needed more water to drink...NO!!! The doctor came in to go over the specifics of the embryo quality with us, it was always a concern that they may not survive the thaw; however, that never happened to us. I don't remember the exact specifics of the embryo but I remember it wasn't great quality. They transfer them in quality order so it was the "worst" of this batch. Kevin got suited up and we headed in. The transfer went just as all the others—there were a couple of students in there that day...as if laying on a sterile table legs spread eagle with a bright light shining on your hoohaa and your husband at one end and the doctor at the other isn't embarrassing enough just add a couple of students to the mix. Laying there on that table I was struggling to hold it together, so many years, so many meds, so much money, so much effort and this was it, this was the end either way it went we were finishing this journey and it was all catching up to me. I was doing all I could do not to break my cardinal rule...no crying in the doctor's office, in fact, I was trying so hard to hold it together and get back behind my curtain before anyone saw a tear fall that I FORGOT to pee!! As I was closing the curtain, Missy asked aren't you going to pee...oh yeah! HAHAHA!!! And just like that, it was over and we headed home...only ever to return to bloodwork and ultrasound if needed, never another retrieval or transfer, it was such a weird feeling. I really felt that day that this part of the journey was over. I 100% knew in my heart that God had great things in store for me, but I did not think they included the success of this day.

JUST WHEN YOU THINK IT'S OVER...THAT'S WHEN IT IS REALLY JUST BEGINNING

～✦～

Facebook post-January 15, 2018: *I posted the link to the song "While I'm Waiting" by John Waller that Jessica had sent me and wrote this: "Someone shared this song with me tonight!! I have heard it many times before, but you better believe when I opened it and played it, I blasted the sound right there in my kitchen and sang like there was no tomorrow (lucky no one was home—for their sake). Waiting is so hard!! Waiting is always hard! Waiting is hard while you're praying, and it's hard while you're putting in the effort and it's especially hard once you've done all you can do except wait (and pray), but in the waiting…that's where the lessons are learned and where the men are separated from the boys (or girls are separated for the women). In the waiting is where we have to TRUST and know that whatever the outcome good things are coming!! After all, Noah had to wait on the flood, Lazarus had to wait to be raised from the dead, Moses had to wait to get out of Egypt and Abraham had to wait to get a son! The wait builds character and courage, my wait has brought me hope and Joy!! The wait can stink sometimes, but I'm thankful for my wait, it has taught me things the outcome never could have! This song is also doubly special tonight because that person sharing it with me tonight is a reminder they are praying for me and wanting the same things I want! So thank you Jessica Rice Moore for the reminder that even in the wait we will praise him! And for the reminder that you are praying for me in the gap when I get tired!! #fightingforjoyandababy #evenwhilewewait #prayingpeoplemakeadifference"*

I was continuing my tradition of thanking God for something with each of my pills, and as tradition went the last one was always reserved for being thankful for that embryo in the freezer in Evansville…but now I was thankful for that embryo snuggled deep in my uterus. As much as I did not think this cycle was going to work, I couldn't help myself from commencing the pee on a stick marathon. And then one morning there it was…the two lines, I didn't believe it, I really, really did not believe this cycle was going to work and I was OK with that and here I was with a positive pregnancy test, after positive pregnancy test. But, I had also been here before and was getting better at that old saying by not letting my highs get too high.

Facebook post-January 19, 2018: "Finding the JOY in a little healthy competition tonight. Friday night of the BIT the only night of the year I still break out the now vintage Sesser shirt. He hates it which is what brings me such joy!! **#findjoyinthelittlethings**"

That's part of how I was getting through this wait…finding the joy in even the smallest of things. That night at that basketball game there was a young couple sitting near us that Kevin knew… and when I say young I would venture to guess they were about 8 or 9 years younger than me. One of Kevin's friends starting giving them a hard time about when they were going to have a baby and it finally came out that they were pregnant, they just weren't telling everyone yet and I was instantly jealous! I was technically pregnant too, I knew that from the 900 tests I had peed on, but I couldn't tell anyone yet and still, in my mind I figured it would end soon, so as much hope and joy as I was fighting for and as much as I was thankful my flesh still showed through at times.

Facebook post-January 21, 2018: *"It is well with my soul."*

Ten days later on January 22, 2018, I had bloodwork drawn on my way to work. I had opted out of going back to the fertility clinic for the blood work as that just really wasn't feasible with my new job, the perk of this was I could see the results on the hospitals my chart system before the doctor's office would call me with results. I was sitting in the library of a small school, next to one of the assistants I work with when I logged in to check the number, by this time I knew the drill…ideally, the number would be well over 100, but anything over 5 meant pregnant, the highest number I had ever had at this point was 160, but then of course that was not successful. And then I saw it on the screen **300!!!** I could not believe my eyes, I think I refreshed the screen 2 or 3 times to make sure I was reading it correctly, and then I spilled my guts to that coworker. Luckily we had known each other for quite a while and she actually knew I was doing this or it could have been an incredibly odd conversation. I immediately texted both Kevin and my mom and then you know what I did? I started googling what could be wrong if that number was too high because there was my flesh shining through, I was doing all I could do to keep my joy and my hope and believe good things were coming for me, but I couldn't stop waiting for the other shoe to fall, waiting for bad things to happen. The doctor's office called that afternoon and assured me that number was great and it did not mean anything was wrong. It would be repeated 48 hours later to ensure a double of the numbers…646!! I was pregnant, at least for now… but then I had been here before…

Messages between Jessica and I

Me: *"So blood test was today. They want the number to be over 100 and the highest number I've ever had at this stage was 160. Number today was 300.8!!! Repeat on Wednesday number needs to double!! Keep those prayers coming. Thank you so much!!"*

Jessica: *"Wow! That's amazing Mariah! I teared up. I will pray for BIG numbers!"*

January 24, 2018

Me: *"646!"*

Jessica: *"Awwwww that is GREAT!! Prayers answered! I'm so excited, I can't stand it. LOL"*

Me: *"Seems as though all is going well. Now we just wait. Ultrasound is scheduled for 2/12"*

Jessica: *"Currently this means you are prego"*

Me: *"Yes ma'am!! Almost 5 weeks"*

Jessica: *"This is great. What is the furthest you have been?"*

Me: *"13 weeks"*

On February 12, 2018, I returned to Evansville for the ultrasound. I had the day off work because of President's day and my mom went with me. I struggled the whole drive of whether she should come in with me...you know just like before, what if there was bad news—remember my no crying rule, but then I thought this is it...no more of these good or bad this is it and why not let her so in we both went. When Missy came to the door to call me back she said a quick prayer with the father, the son and the holy ghost and I thanked her for that…she knew we needed all the prayers we could get. Missy also knew me enough to know not to beat around the bush…there were other things that had to be looked at and measured but she was quick to find it and quick to point out that heartbeat… and there it was again only this time x 2…my mom and I both took a deep breath. She proceeded with all her measurements and calculations and then Doctor Griffin started giving me his spiel…and this is the telltale sign of the infertility clinic if Dr. Griffin talks to you in that room it is good news, if he has you get dressed and come to the office it is bad news…we got to talk in the ultrasound room today!! Dr. Griffin gave me the choice of getting lab work done the next couple of weeks at my local hospital or returning for lab work and ultrasounds, but we both agreed there was no need for the ultrasounds, as I knew that it really didn't matter, there was nothing they could do to stop whatever was going to happen until later. I walked out that day done…never to come back to this place again, I felt like I had become a constant there, we had been there longer than most of the office staff, I knew that office and that routine like the back of my hand and I was done whatever this outcome (I would go back one more time, but more on that later).

NOT MAKING THE SAME MISTAKE AS LAST TIME, IN MORE THAN ONE WAY

At the beginning of February, I was officially released from the infertility doc and could go to my own OB. The day of my previous miscarriage I had actually called a new office because I felt I wasn't getting the care I needed, so my plan was to return to that practice this time. I was not stepping foot back in the office from last time. When I called the new office I had a couple of stipulations, I wanted seen at least once by them before I was released so they could talk with Dr. Griffin and I wanted to only see one doctor every time I went. That's not how they usually do it, but I convinced them and they allowed it and I will forever be grateful for that. I wanted someone that knew me and knew my story, I needed someone to fight for this baby as much as I was! On February 16, 2018, Kevin and I went for our first appointment with a new doctor, this was sort of an informal visit, no tests today just a history and meeting each other. So we went through our whole story with him and made it clear we were nervous, we were scared, we were hopeful and we needed help! I remember him saying to us that we were a scary case to take on and the only thing he knew to do was to turn it over to God and to pray about it...ahh, a man after our own hearts! He was also super understanding of my crazy mind and agreed to bi-weekly ultrasounds to ensure all was going well.

Facebook post-February 16, 2018: *I posted a memory from 6 years ago that said "I do not have to know why everything happens since I know God is good, he loves me and life on Earth is not the whole story" and wrote this: "4 years old and truer today than the day I wrote it. This has been a big part of my attitude change over the last year and a big help in my fight for joy. My new mantra is that I know good things are coming!!! I don't know what they are, I know what I would like them to be and what I hope they are, but I also know if those things don't work out that it's ok because good things ARE coming!! Some of my favorite verses in the Bible have to do with God giving us the desires of our heart, but I think for a long time I interpreted those incorrectly I used to think there's no way he could give everyone the desires of their heart because everyone's doesn't match up… but I think I was being too superficial, too shallow I have some things I want, but the true desires of my heart are things like happiness, hope and joy and sometimes I may come about those things differently than I originally thought, but ultimately he will give me those true desires if I will trust him and let his plan work!! So here's to good things (my good things and your good things), whatever they may be because they ARE coming!!" #fightingforjoyandababy*

So I was going to the doctor every 2 weeks for an ultrasound and to check in with him and all was going well!! We made it past the 8-week mark which is the week they found the subchorionic hematoma before and all was still looking great!!

I don't remember the exact date, but I remember it was in the evening. We had finished supper and clean up and were just chilling watching TV, I went to the bathroom to pee and when I wiped… there it was blood (spotting) on the toilet paper…see I knew it, this was not going to work. I actually thought I held it together pretty good, but Kevin would later talk about the look on my face when I came out of the bathroom that night, as terrible, the saddest thing he had ever seen and he never wanted to see it again. I knew from experience that nothing could be done that night so I waited until the next morning to call the doctor, they got me in for an ultrasound and I heard the tech say these words, "there is a small bleed", and I lost it!! She kept reassuring me that the baby looked good and the bleed was small and I just kept telling her I had heard all that before—the Nurse practitioner came in to talk to me and again tried to reassure me they were common and would likely go away, but I just kept telling them they didn't understand, we had been here before. They sent me home on pelvic rest (basically no sex) and stopped my aspirin, which is two things they did not do last time, so at least I felt like we were doing something different.

Facebook post-February 22, 2018: *I posted a picture/memory from the night Kevin proposed to me in 2014 and wrote this: "This memory popped up on Facebook from 4 years ago…oh what a memory it is! Look at those babies!! Oh, we were so naïve. I answered one of the most important questions of my life that night and I have never regretted the answer. Now don't get me wrong, there have been some times when it has been a struggle and our 4 years have not been always great but I wouldn't want to do life with anyone else. We vowed, in the beginning, to keep God in the center of our marriage and I'm so thankful every day that he's there. Oh what a memory from that Sonic parking lot 4 years ago, here's to 50 more Kevin Stubblefield!"*

I went in for an ultrasound on a Friday afternoon in March, they were still doing ultrasounds twice a week to monitor the bleeds, the ultrasound tech's exact words were that things were hard to see because my uterus was messy. She never came out and said it but I think things looked bad that day. She just called it messy and reiterated several times to me what to do in case I had bleeding over the weekend. She did tell me that the bleeds were still small and baby looked good, but I remember again she told me where and how to seek help if I had bleeding over the weekend. I don't think I grasped how concerned she was until I went in for my next ultrasound the following Monday and she seemed so relieved that baby was safe and my uterus was no longer "messy". We were getting close to the 12-week mark but of course, we had been there before and it didn't mean much, but it was getting increasingly difficult to keep it a secret.

On March 28th—I went in for an ultrasound—Kevin went with me and I remember saying to Jackie that I knew no one knew with 100% certainty how any pregnancy would turn out, let alone one of mine, but I asked her if she felt like the bleeds were small enough and were being absorbed enough that we could let the cat out of the bag? It shocked me when she said yes! Medical professionals are usually so non-committal but she never wavered. Kevin and I discussed it on the way home and decided we were ready to spill our guts!

Becoming public once again!

When we got home from the ultrasound that night I was going to make a post on Facebook, but it was harder than I thought. The last time we did this we quickly regretted it and I was afraid for a repeat, I was also just afraid for people to know...I don't know why no one was anything but ecstatic for us but it was nerve-wracking none the less.

Facebook post-March 28, 2018: "If at first, you don't succeed... try again, pray again, believe again, hope again and most of all keep your joy!! We've been nervously excited for several weeks now, but it's time to let the cat out of the bag! Baby Stubblefield due September 2018!! It has been a journey! Thank you for all the prayers that have been said on our behalf and feel free to keep them coming!"

Later that week someone in a meeting at work asked me if I was a parent and I said "No but I will be in September" and that was the first time I had really "told" someone with my voice and the first time I brought it up at work—where people had no idea what I had been doing. It was a milestone of sorts and coming out—so to speak!!

Facebook post-March 30, 2018 (Easter Weekend): *"It is well with my soul. "It is finished"—I am so thankful for this weekend. Without what happened this weekend thousands of years ago we would not have the promise of Heaven. I am thankful for God's plan then and now. A large part of my heart lives in Heaven, and because Jesus was crucified for my sins and rose again, I get to go there some-day! I feel like this weekend can also remind us that our situations can change in an instant. Jesus was DEAD and rose again!! And sometimes things in our life may die (our hopes, our dreams, our joy) but they can rise again in Jesus! If you read my posts at all you know I am currently in the upswing of life and for that, I am beyond grateful, but I have had times when I was not in the upswing...but in those times Jesus STILL died for me (and for you)!! Take the time this weekend to reflect on what Jesus did for our benefit and as always find some joy this Easter! "Up from the grave, he arose!"*

The next time we had an ultrasound the tech told us she thought at the next visit she would be able to tell the sex of the baby—so we brought both our moms to that appointment...a moment I will never forget—she searched and searched my belly for what seemed like forever before she said OK I'm certain it's a GIRL!!! And at that moment I knew I would have a best friend for the rest of my life!!!! She also told us at that visit that they could no longer find the bleeds—and it was also at that moment that I felt like maybe we were going to make it after all!

Facebook post-April 4, 2018: *"These things I have spoken to you, that my joy may be in you and that your joy may be full"—John 15:11. Our joy is certainly full today!! Let the shoes and bows and clothes begin! Baby Stubblefield is a GIRL, most importantly baby is HEALTHY! Thank you again for all the prayers!!!"*

LIVING LIFE PREGNANT!!

~~~~~~

I counted down the days to the ultrasounds—seeing the baby and hearing the heartbeat was a feeling I cannot explain. A sense of relief beyond any other, but it never lasted long. Things were going well, for the most part, aside from the bleeds which were gone, and yet I still worried every second of every day that something would go wrong. If ever a person lived by the book it was me, no diet soda, no caffeine, no lifting, pelvic rest, no lunchmeat, no soft cheese—if a book anywhere or the internet said it could be harmful to a pregnancy, I didn't do it and yet I still worried this was going to end any second. As strongly as I believed good things were coming and knew without a shadow of a doubt that God had this under control I still didn't believe this was going to work out—it is such an odd feeling to explain. At one of our early on visits with the OB, he mentioned that I had PTSD, and I believe he was right. All I could ever think about was all the things that had gone wrong before and all the things that could go wrong—I was in a constant state of panic, prayer and excitement!! I was continuing my nightly routine of thanking God with each of my pills; however, that last one had changed—we had progressed now from thanking God for the embryo in the freezer in Indiana to thanking god for the fetus snuggled up in my uterus, and now thanking God for that little girl growing inside of me!

Facebook post-April 19, 2018: *I posted a picture of my brother and wrote this: "I could have missed the pain but I'd have to miss the dance" —Garth Brooks 13 years ago tomorrow this guy got to go* *"home". I can't imagine what it must be like to stroll the streets of gold or to experience the peace that comes when you look into Jesus' face. When I think of it from my earthly point of view, I think about all he has missed…but I'm sure he isn't missing anything as he is far better where he is. 13 years ago I remember being terrified of what life would bring now, I bet I asked my parents 150 times in the 24 hours after he died if we were going to be ok, and I remember being terrified to sleep or be in a room by myself, but life moves on and we learn to dance again. I wouldn't trade the dance for anything…the key… enjoy the dance while you're dancing because the music could stop in the blink of an eye! Fight for joy, keep dancing and know where you're going when it's over! See you on the other side, Christopher."*

Last time I was pregnant I had bought some maternity clothes and I think I had even worn a pair of maternity pants one time (it was early but hey I wanted to do it so bad!), but in April of 2018, I really started wearing maternity clothes, took my first "bump" picture and someone told me they could tell I was pregnant. These are all milestones I never thought I would reach!!

Facebook post-May 1, 2018: *"Before I formed you in the womb I knew you before you were born I set you apart; I appointed you as a prophet to the nations."—Jeremiah 1:5 If you want proof God exists…here it is!! The top picture is Baby girl Stubblefield (yes she is still nameless!) as a 6-day old embryo after being in the freezer for 9 months, the bottom Is what she looks like today! How you can go from one to the other is AMAZING!! God is Real! God is Awesome! We are full of JOY! She is our miracle!!" **#Fullofjoy #Godisreal***

On May 13, 2018, I celebrated my second Mother's Day; however, I didn't celebrate at all. The year before I was pregnant with our little boy and we weren't "public" but Kevin and I knew and I remember at the very end of the day he told me Happy Mother's Day—and I felt like yes Happy Mother's Day to me and well… we all know how that ended. This year I was most definitely pregnant and "out" and many, many people wished me a "Happy Mother's Day" and my response was always I am not a mom yet—such a false statement for so so many reasons. The very first time I stepped foot into that fertility clinic I was a mom, when I endured that AWFUL HSG test I was a mom, every hoohaa ultrasound I endured, and every shot I took in my butt I was a mom! I was a mom to multiple children I will never get to hold on this side of paradise and yet I was afraid if I acknowledged this as a Mother's Day it would all come crashing down. I promise I had faith and hope during this time and I was beyond full of Joy but it was a constant battle within myself to not assume the worst at all times.

Facebook post-May 13, 2018: *I posted a couple "pictures" on Facebook that read "On Mother's Day I can think of no mother more deserving than a mother that had to give one back." –Erma Bombeck, "This is a mother who would do anything for her baby…even before conception has taken place.", and "Faith in God includes faith in His timing" and wrote this: "Just a friendly reminder…today is HARD for some people! I am beyond grateful and blessed that I am on this side this year but that has not always been the case. There are grieving mothers out there who have lost children, there are women that have spent thousands of dollars, countless hours and taken many a shot who still don't have a child and women who would give everything they had to be celebrated today and while mothers stick out to them always—today it is thrown in their face…today they are reminded what they are not…so be kind for today is a hard battle for many people. "The Lord is close to the brokenhearted and saves those that are crushed in spirit" –Psalm 34:18"*

Shortly after Mother's Day comes Father's Day of course and as much as I battled the uncharted territory that was Mother's Day, Father's Day was even worse for Kevin—last year on Father's Day we were "out" 100%, he was wished Happy Father's Day by multiple people and I made a Facebook post about it, I had even gotten him a knife as a gift—the knife that would later be placed in the "casket" with our little boy—Kevin wanted no part of Father's Day until he was holding his little girl in his arms. Kevin too was a father the very first time he rolled into that clinic, he was a father with both miserable procedures, he was a father every time he comforted a sad wife and every time he gave a shot. Father's Day went mostly unnoticed in our house this year—I missed my dad more than anyone can imagine and Kevin wasn't ready.

APPRECIATING NEW THINGS

꧁ ꧂

Facebook post-June 19, 2018: *I posted a picture of the OB waiting room and this saying "I still remember the days I prayed for the things I have now." And posted this: "Today I'm spending my morning sitting in a waiting room for 3 hours...(the dreaded 3-hour glucose test...though it has not been as bad as I feared), at first I was aggravated. Who wants to sit for 3 hours...then I remembered. I remembered how long I have wanted this. For 3 years I fought to get to this waiting room (and when you think about that, 3 hours is nothing compared to 3 years). I have spent countless hours in waiting rooms, some in Illinois, some in Missouri, some in Indiana and some in Kentucky waiting for bloodwork, waiting for procedures, waiting for doctors and while remarkably they all are so similar...flowered carpet, plastic chairs and ALWAYS HGTV on the tv (I guess they figure that's what hormonal women want to watch)...this waiting room right here this is the one I've been fighting for—the one where I rest my hands on my bump while I wait, the one where I'm no longer jealous of the pregnant women around me but I am the pregnant one, the one where I won't be crying when I leave. I remember those 3 years of waiting rooms most like they were yesterday, and I remember how hard I've prayed and fought to get here, and while I sit here for these 3 hours I am no longer aggravated, I am happy. This, this is what I wanted. Sometimes we get caught up in life and we forget we are right where we wanted to be. This will likely be a one-time experience for me (and I am perfectly fine with that) and I am going to savor it, I'm going to soak it in...this, this waiting room for 3 hours, this is right where I wanted to be! Keep praying, keep fight-*

ing and remember to stop sometimes and enjoy where you are."
#winningthefightforjoyandababy

It is interesting how the struggle to get pregnant and then finally experiencing a pregnancy changed my perspective on so many things. The things many other people take for granted or complain about are things I fought for and truly tried to savor. In June it was though my life had come full circle from that ER room where the nurse was wiping the blood as it ran down my legs to soaking up the baby kicks and growing belly!

Facebook post-June 28, 2018: *"I debated whether or not to post anything today…I'm flying pretty high right now and no one wants to mix sadness and joy…but the truth is they are always mixed so I decided to go ahead. 1 year ago today we were pretty close to rock bottom…1 year ago today we lost our son (I never really know how to say that, technically it was a miscarriage but that doesn't seem harsh enough, I saw him, perfectly formed, not a fetus at all just a very small baby, he was picked up at the hospital by the funeral home and he is buried in a cemetery) and our story became public, we began a public fight for joy and a baby. I remember the days following that loss…Kevin and I went through the time I call drowning our sorrows in material items. I never want to forget this little boy, he taught me so much about myself, about Kevin and about God. It's strange to think about him now because if things would have gone differently we probably wouldn't be where we are right now (and we are in a pretty good place right now), but I do know he paved the way for His sister. I actually had the same problem earlier in this pregnancy that I had with him, and because of him they knew how to treat it this time, so without him, we would not have her…she is our comeback. Out of the ashes, we rose! A year ago if someone would have told me we would be here today I don't know if I would have understood the*

joy we would have. So much can change in a year (really...so much can change in an instant)...this is the message I want to give today... DO NOT dwell on your current circumstances...they can change!!! If we would have got stuck last year, where would we be now?... we would be sad and broke (remember the indulgence into material things haha) but we didn't get stuck we grew so so much closer, Kevin was my rock, we grew stronger and we clung to God because we knew he was still in control!!! We fought hard this year for joy and a baby and her picture is below...she is our Joy! I will never forget my little boy...but I will not get stuck in grief. Instead I will know I will see him again one day and I will enjoy where I am now... who knows what this year will bring. Remember do not get stuck in your current circumstances, they CAN change! Keep fighting for what you want and keep fighting for Joy! Life is fragile (I was reminded of that even this week) so enjoy it! Your comeback is coming!!!!
#winningthefightforjoyandababy

PREPARING WITH CAUTION

That summer was full of preparations, primarily nursery preparations, cleaning out the spare bedroom and preparing it to be the nursery, preparing ourselves to be parents and changing our mindset. Even as we grew closer to the due date and the need to prepare became real it was still scary to me. I'm not a superstitious person and I don't believe in circumstance or curse or anything like that, I believe in God and his goodness and that he has it all under control but I still felt like if I let it become too real it would vanish. I guess it was taking Kevin's words of advice to heart about not letting my highs get too high. My mom and I took a big shopping trip in July that summer to Nashville and I remember as we walked out of the first baby store after making a purchase I said to my mom "well she just kicked so I guess she's still alive" and my mom said something like oh Mariah you can't think like that and then she said but you notice that's the first big purchase I've made. Don't get me wrong we had of course been preparing (for years really) but nervously.

Facebook post-July 31, 2018: *I posted a picture of my Grandpa and wrote this: "It's getting real up in here!! 61 days to the due date... just wow!! It's hard to believe after all the work and time it has taken to get here and it is really happening. We have been on nursery prep for a while around the Stubblefield house, but this man right here has been on nursery prep even longer than us. When we first started trying to have a baby we talked to him about building us a crib, and he never doubted and he never wavered. He knew he would build us one someday and today...today it was delivered and it is*

119

GORGEOUS!! Besides the work he put into this crib, I also know he has put countless prayers into me and Maddie. I'm so thankful for him and everything he means to me, and not many people can say their 80-year-old grandpa build their baby's crib! Love you, Grandpa!!"

I truly believe my grandpa never doubted he would build me this crib. We always joke that he plans projects in his head 100 times before he executes them and I know he never stopped planning that crib and I also know that he said countless prayers for me and my baby, it not only takes a village to raise a child but it took a village to get me a child!

The rest of the summer brought more excitement and baby prep. On August 3rd, 2018 I celebrated my baby shower!! A day I wasn't sure I would ever experience! At the end of this summer is also when my thankful prayers took their final shift and the lion sleeper made its final move. With my pills each night my last pill had been reserved from day one for that little embryo in the freezer and then changed to the embryo nestled in my uterus, to the baby in my uterus, to the little girl in my belly and then finally to thanking God for Maddie! Also, the lion sleeper made its final move as it was washed and packed in the hospital bag. Kevin insisted it be the first thing Maddie wore in the hospital. I balked a little just because it kind of looked like a boy outfit, but Kevin insisted saying he looked at it empty for 3 years and was tired of seeing it that way and it would be the first thing she wore, so I searched for and purchased a green bow to match!

Facebook post-August 26, 2018: *"Then Jesus said, "Did I not tell you, that if you believe, you will see the Glory of God" –John 11:40. The finishing touch was put on the nursery tonight, all the necessities* *have been bought, bags are beginning to be packed...this is really happening. We are bringing home a baby. As I sit here tonight and look around this room, I can't help but remember when I bought the very first baby outfit, and then when we began "stocking up," and now look at this room, it is ready for a baby...MY BABY. I feel truly blessed beyond measure when I look around this room, I see beds that were made and purchased by people who already love Maddie, I see clothes and blankets made for her by people who prayed right along with us through this whole season, I see a room fit for my miracle. I know some people are probably getting tired of hearing about our story or quite frankly our happy ending, which I understand (when you're in the battle, you can get very tired of hearing other people's happy ending...and p.s. that does NOT make you a bad person), but I also know that Maddie is a true modern-day miracle, and her story is important! Faith can move mountains and faith brought me Maddie and people need to know that. I'm not going to lie, when I hear about people getting pregnant on a whim or on a first try part of me still goes crazy on the inside, it's crazy to me that people can make babies from one night stands, or on an impulse in the backseat of a car...my baby took meticulous calculations, embryologists, doctors, countless procedures and tubes of blood, my baby came at a cost both financial and emotional but then I remember, I remember everything this journey taught me...those things are secrets those people will never know. My baby took work, and faith and more love than you could ever imagine. I learned to trust God when it looks like it will never happen, I learned that God has his own way of doing things and we can't second guess that. I learned that faith takes work, perseverance and I learned that sometimes with the very last ounce of faith you have you buy the diapers for the baby you won't have for 2 more years. I want people to know that God is still in the prayer answering business and I want people to know that you have to fight for what you want! I do hope Maddie's story reaches people, and I hope that whatever you're wanting or needing tonight that you keep the faith and you know that your miracle is coming, maybe not how or when you want it to come, but it IS coming. "Therefore I tell you, whatever you ask for in prayer, believe that you have received it, and it will be yours" —Mark 11:24"* **#winningthefightforjoyandababy**

BABY MONTH

Facebook post-September 1, 2018: *I posted a memory from the previous year and wrote this: "This post came up on my memories today…there are so many things to say about this post. First I still miss this guy something fierce and wish so so much he could be here right now! Second, this post is 100% proof that your circumstances can change! I posted this one year ago…I lost my job that day, I was fighting so hard to have a baby and I was scared!! Fast forward 365 days…I LOVE my new job! I was blessed to be off all summer and I am blessed to work with some awesome people. And it is BABY MONTH! One year…so so much can happen and change in one year! It will be exciting to see what this next year holds!"*

Early September was relatively uneventful, people were starting to make wagers on when Maddie would arrive. I remember leaving work one day in the very beginning of September and a coworker asked my due date and when I responded he said, "but you're hoping sooner right?" and I remember saying "No, not really I'm doing good!" and I meant that. I was getting excited of course but I really wasn't ready for it to be over. While I was getting excited Kevin was getting nervous! He talked a lot about making sure we got to the hospital in time, I wasn't so worried about that, I knew it didn't really happen like the movies depicted and we would have time to get there but that was his main fear! On September 1ˢᵗ—I went to breakfast with my grandparents and aunts and uncles, I remember my grandma wanting everyone to take their guess of my due date, I don't remember all the guesses, but I remember my grandpa went with October 1ˢᵗ since that was his birthday and my Grandma went with September 13th—and I remember thinking goodness Grandma that is soon! HAHAHA.

SEPTEMBER 10, 2018

It was a Monday like any other Monday, I saw a kiddo for the first time that school year that day—his mom was there and made a comment to me about the baby and saying now that I had seen him I could go ahead and have my baby and I remember thinking not yet, it's too early!

That night Kevin got home later in the evening following football practice and as he was coming in he said to me, "I have to get a picture, you have gotten a lot bigger today." He constantly commented on my size during the pregnancy and I would joke that that was not a nice thing to say, but he always reminded me it was a good thing because it meant our baby was healthy and growing. He took a "bump" picture that night because he just couldn't get over what he felt like was the difference from morning to night. I remember I had made a cake the night before just because and ate a piece after supper. I commented to Kevin that it tasted weird-like I had used too much butter or something because it felt weird in my mouth.

As had been Kevin's main fear for a while now we talked about getting to the hospital. He expressed that he was worried about getting there in time and did not want to go multiple times just to be sent home. He proceeded to say a very specific prayer—he prayed specifically that he would KNOW when it was time to go to the hospital. He prayed that there would be no guessing that we would just know to go, that we would not be sent home and that we would have plenty of time. Be careful what you pray for!

I would later joke with him that maybe he should have specified some other things and that I wasn't sure I wanted him praying for me!!

SEPTEMBER 11, 2018

I had been having some trouble sleeping and would wake up early in the morning and be unable to go back to sleep. I woke up around 5 am that morning and couldn't go back to sleep so I thought I would go ahead and take my shower then lay back down so that's what I did. When I got up again to get ready I went into the bathroom to brush my teeth, but when I went to swish with the water I couldn't keep it in my mouth. It was bizarre! I would swish and it would just roll out, I think I tried 3 or 4 times before I looked in the mirror and when I did I thought that's weird my mouth looks funny. I smiled and could tell my mouth was not moving right. I proceeded to check some other things, opening and closing my eyes, sticking my tongue out and such and then went in the bedroom to see what Kevin thought. I said, "Does my face look funny to you?" and I looked up at him and smiled...he went into panic mode! He said, "YES it does, we are going to the ER." I told him to calm down and take a picture so I could send it to my mom—it wouldn't be till later when I looked at that picture that I realized how bad I looked that morning. Kevin was worried I was having a stroke, but I had already assessed by upper extremity strength and ROM and knew my cognition was intact—I really wasn't worried about that but Kevin was. He got ready the fastest I have ever seen that morning. My mom suggested we either go to the ER or to the doctor's office—Kevin wanted me in the ER—NOW!!! As we were leaving we decided to take the baby bag, just in case.

I'm not exactly sure how fast Kevin drove that day on the way to the ER, but I know it certainly wasn't the speed limit! When we arrived at the ER, they called up to OB to decide where we should go, since I was so pregnant normally a person would go straight to OB, but since my complaint wasn't really pregnancy related they weren't sure, but ultimately decided to send me to OB. When I got into the room and told them my complaint of facial droop and smiled the nurse said, "well, I can see that!" They got me in bed and hooked me up to monitors where I would stay for the rest of the day. It was relatively relaxed. Kevin and my mom were there, we didn't really call anyone else yet because we weren't sure what was happening. They ordered an ultrasound and Kevin's best friend came in to do that which was kind of neat—everything looked great!

When the doctor came in that afternoon he checked my cervix, I was 4 cm dilated and was contracting but they weren't strong—he decided to wait a little while and call a specialist to decide what to do. I was 37 weeks and 2 days pregnant so I could have the baby—but they really didn't want to induce just because yet. When he came back later he said the specialist advised induction. I was experiencing bell's palsy—which was my assumption and this can sometimes be an early warning sign of preeclampsia, which I was already being watched for and my blood pressure was elevated. His exact words were "we have nothing to gain and everything to lose by keeping you pregnant"—valid point Dr. Asberry, valid point!

And so, at 5:00 p.m. on September 11, 2018, my induction began. Many visitors started trickling in—Kevin's mom and sister, my grandparents and lots of friends because of course Kevin worked there! Also, our preacher showed up that evening and as if to come full circle—he stood there at the head of my bed, arms and legs crossed and looked at me—much like he had that day in December 2017—of course, his look was much different this time!!

I had told Kevin all along that I wanted to try to do labor without an epidural—it's weird I know but I guess I thought since this would likely never happen again I wanted to experience every bit of it and I just thought it would sound cool and tough to tell people I did it without an epidural—but after they broke my water that went out the window and I asked for the epidural!! When I got the epidural everyone had to leave the room—it was just me, the nurse and the anesthesiologist—WOW!! Infertility and childbirth, in general, are a humbling experience but the epidural was rough! I needed help sitting up, I hurt so bad I was crying—the nurse was holding me the anesthesiologist was telling me not to move—I got nauseous and puked—I felt so bad for that nurse, I think I apologized ten times. After the epidural, I was able to get some rest before it was time to push.

Pushing was HARD—It really didn't hurt because my epidural was working so good—in fact maybe too good and at one point they did have to turn it off, but it was just hard work—I pushed for almost 2 hours. You would think at this point we would all feel pretty confident about the outcome but that is not the case. My mom became very worried during the pushing that something would happen to me and actually had to sit down for a little while, and part of me was still worried she would come out not breathing—that PTSD, that idea that bad things happen a lot was hard to shake even right there in the delivery room.

At 2:56 AM on September 12, 2018, Maddie Joy Stubblefield entered the world! I think I asked 20 times in her first minute of life why she wasn't crying and if she was ok. The doctor kept telling me he hadn't stimulated her yet and not to borrow trouble and the nurse kept telling me I would know if something was wrong that they would not be that calm. When I heard her cry and they placed her on my chest—that's when I took the first deep breath in 3 years! I had just delivered a healthy baby girl! She had 10 fingers and 10 toes and a full head of dark hair—she was pure perfection!!

Facebook post-September 12, 2018: *"You turned my wailing into dancing; you removed my sackcloth and clothed me with JOY"* *—Psalm 30: 11 "Maddie Joy Stubblefield made her entrance at 2:56 AM September 12, 2018, and she is PERFECT. 6lbs 11 oz 20 in long. I still cannot believe this is real. We fought for her!! We continue to be so so grateful for all the prayers said on our behalf. She truly is a miracle and truly is our JOY. With Jesus' help, we beat infertility's butt!!!"* ***#wewonthefightforjoyandababy***

WHEN YOU THOUGHT YOU CONQUERED JOY—BUT YOU'RE SAD

For several weeks at every doctor's appointment, my OB had been warning me about becoming sad after I had Maddie. Every time he talked about it my thoughts were...yeah right, do you know how hard I've worked for this, how much I want this?? I will not be sad!!— Well turns out there's a reason he's a doctor and I'm not. Shortly after coming home from the hospital with Maddie, the sadness hit.

I was unable to breastfeed Maddie. I tried really, really hard. I thought I was doing good—Maddie seemed perfectly content. When we went to Maddie's first doctor's appointment she had lost over a pound and she was jaundiced. Our pediatrician was blunt and told me either we started some formula or Maddie was going to end up back in the hospital. So for the next several days Maddie was on bili lights and I would attempt to nurse her for 10-20 minutes on each side, then feed her formula, then pump to see what I could get—which was never more than half an ounce and that was rare. When we returned to the doctor, Maddie's numbers were better from the formula and the lights but I was sad. Our pediatrician gave me some very good words of wisdom. She could sense my sadness over not being able to breastfeed and she said breastfeeding is limited—maybe a year-long and after that, all babies eat the same things anyway—it isn't worth missing the here and now and stressing over it—you're missing these early days of enjoyment with your baby. She was so right!! I was letting that little thing steal my joy!

I have missed my dad every day since he died and I imagine I always will—but those first few days and weeks after Maddie arrived were rough—I felt so so much like he needed to be there! When I looked at her face it just hurt deep in my heart to know he would never meet or hold my sweet Maddie girl on this side of Heaven. I have since warned people I know that have lost a parent and are expecting a baby that they will miss that parent more than ever before. This was stealing my joy!

Along with not being able to breastfeed and missing my dad like crazy I was so sad to not be pregnant anymore. It's hard to explain—I fought so hard for a baby and wanted it so bad and here I had it and I was sad! It was just so final to think I would never be pregnant again, never wear maternity clothes again, never feel the baby kick inside me again, never have another ultrasound, never labor again and never bring another life into this world. Also, my face was still recovering from the bell's palsy—I couldn't use a straw, I was struggling to use a spoon, when I yawned or cried one side of my face tightened up and then it just got me more upset…I was struggling.

I remember saying to Kevin during one of my break down moments—people must think I'm crazy! I have this perfectly perfect little baby that I so desperately wanted and I was sad…but I truly believe that was the devil trying to steal my joy. I remember going to my two-week follow-up and my OB asked about the sadness—I was doing a little better by this point but I told him he was right it had hit for sure. I often wondered and still do at times, if I didn't have these extenuating circumstances if I still would have been sad. The main things making me sad were not common and I wonder if they weren't there if I would have just found something else to be sad about. Those first couple of weeks were and always will be a reminder to me that the devil is always trying to steal your joy! Even if you feel like you have conquered it, like you own the joy, you have to be careful because he is still lurking!

It is also hard to explain but following Maddie's birth I felt like my relationship with God was struggling. Trying to get to Maddie, carrying Maddie and birthing Maddie had brought me so close to God—we talked about those things all day every day for years—and now she was here and I felt like some of my closeness was gone—I know that probably doesn't make a lot of sense but it is something I have really had to work on and am still working on to get that close relationship back with God.

Once I moved on from the breastfeeding and we got in a rhythm with the bottles and formula and my face gradually got better, I started to miss my dad a little less and continued to just try to soak up every second with Maddie!

A GLIMPSE AT THE FIRST YEAR

◁∼◿

Facebook post from Kevin September 23, 2018: *"This was a special day that was 3 years in the making, with lots of trials and tribulations. We had some great Drs. Dr. Schrepferman and Dr. Griffin set up the meeting and we are forever grateful to them, but God gave us this life. Almost 4 years ago we were married at this alter and it has been a heck of a ride. Now today we stood at this alter to give back to God what he gave to us. Today was Maddie's baby dedication. So many tiny details had to work and go together for Maddie to get here, and when there is a design like that there is a designer. Maddie truly is a miracle baby and she will be raised to know where she came from…faith and prayer."*

Facebook post-September 26, 2018: *"The last 2 weeks have been a whirlwind and have left me speechless!! "Every good and perfect gift is from above…"—James 1:17. Maddie is beyond perfect…3 years of waiting, multiple losses, hundreds if not thousands of shots and you know what…it was ALL worth it, it all had a purpose and truly none of it matters now! I would do it all again for her, I would do it all 100 ties for her…and God knew that the whole time!! God knew what was coming for me…God created Maddie for Kevin and me. Sometimes we just stare at her and think of the goodness of God!! Someday I will go into more detail about the last 2 weeks, there are so many details that reveal the goodness of God and a few details that remind me that even in extreme love and excitement the devil will try to steal your joy, but he will not win! We are so in awe of God's work and so so in love!! Prepare yourself for picture overload…I can't help myself!! "And we know that in all things God works for* *the good of those who love him and have been called according to his purpose" —Romans 8:28"* **#wewonthefightforjoyandababy #Jesusandthestubblefieldskickedinfertilitysbutt**

October 6, 2018: *I shared the story of the elephant and dog being pregnant together again and wrote this: "I've shared this before but it's so true and perfect I have to share it every time I see it. What I carried is "mighty and great." People look at her in admiration and when my baby was born the Earth felt it!! I know it's easy for me to say now, as I'm on the other side as I'm typing this with a sleeping baby on my chest but I am thankful for our journey. Though it was HARD and LONG, I carried and birthed a great thing. I overheard someone call her a miracle baby today and that she is. Maddie and her story will reach people I would never be able to reach. My baby will do great things!!"*

October 15, 2018: (National pregnancy and infant loss awareness day) *"I will always remember the journey we went on, and I will see my babies again one day, but I will never dwell in the grief. God knew what he was doing the whole time!"*

October 19, 2018: *"I have fought the good fight, I have finished the race, I have kept the faith." —2 Timothy 4:7. Today was the equivalent of the victory lap in NASCAR races. I can't even begin to fathom a guess of how many trips I made to Evansville. I would say well over 100 is a safe guess. Some by myself, some with Kevin, some with my mom and few I treasure the most now are the few I made with my dad (he was part of this journey even if he didn't get to see the outcome). Most of the trips were made in the wee early hours of the morning…when I sit and think back on them I can remember most of them. When you sit to have your blood drawn in this office you can see a portion of this wall….I stared that wall down hun-*

dreds of times…I memorized the names you could see and I thought about the day Kevin and I could experience this…and there we are (p.s. I made sure Maddie's footprint is visible from the blood draw chair). When we started this journey in September of 2015, I would say there were less than 50 footprints on this wall…as it grew and grew I often wondered if we would ever joint it. The last couple of pictures are of a new wing that was added to this hospital…the ortho and neuro hospital…when we started going there they had not even started it and now it is finished. They built a hospital and we built a baby. We will forever be grateful for Dr. Griffin and everyone at Boston IVF. They were wonderful!!"

October 29, 2018: *"one day you'll be staring at the blessing you used to always dream about. This is my life right now!!!!"*

November 2, 2018: *"Maddie attended her first girls night tonight. I love these 2 girls! Sometimes our lives get crazy busy and we don't see each other for a while but when we do we pick right up where we left off. When you're fighting for things and your joy, it's important to have good friends fighting beside you. I will always always be thankful for the job that introduced us to each other. These girls were with me through it all and they were the first people besides family to know about Maddie. It did my heart good to see them hold her tonight! They prayed for her just like I did. I'm so glad Maddie will have them in her life. Strong, smart women are great role models. Love you guys!!"*

November 7, 2018: *I posted a picture of Maddie and a picture of my brother and wrote this: "I don't know how I ever lived without this!! Today at this moment I am reminded that grief and JOY can coexist!! I'm gonna say it again for the people in the back…grief and JOY can coexist!! My brother would have been 33 today, but instead,* *he will be forever 19. He is no more or less gone today than any other day but I remember him a little extra on his birthday and I think about all he would have missed this year. I'm sure he would have been a great uncle! I will always have grief, we all have grief of some kind. My life has had a lot of loss, but oh it has had a lot of joy. As I sit here holding my sweet miracle I am full of JOY! So the lesson here is to always find the joy, you can have grief and sadness and anger but you can't get stuck, you must always continue fighting for joy. So as I remember my brother a little extra today I am just doubly reminded to enjoy what life we have because it can be over in the blink of an eye. So happy birthday Bubby!!! I'll see you again someday in paradise."*

November 12, 2018: *" Where did my tiny newborn baby go?!?!?! Maddie is 2 months old today! What a 2 months it has been! She is the BEST baby. She smiles all the time and sleeps 7 hours at night. Every time I look at her I think how blessed I am. She was worth every shot, every doctor's appointment and every bit of the struggle. I wouldn't trade her for the world. My days off with her are dwindling, so I'm soaking up every second of baby snuggles."*

November 21, 2018: *"Every year at this time instead of doing the everyday thankful posts, I usually compile a list…but this year it's different!! This year Maddie tops that list and really fills every space! So I decided to do a list of the things I'm thankful for about Maddie and our journey to get her. I do want to mention though I am so so thankful for many things not just Maddie, including Jesus who died for my sins and my family (I couldn't make a thankful post without including those 2 for sure!). so here goes the 2018 thankful list of Maddie!! I am thankful for/that*

1) *She is a healthy baby!!*
2) *She sleeps at night!*

3) *She is happy almost all the time!*

4) *All the prayers that were said on our behalf during our journey to Maddie.*

5) *We were financially, emotionally and physically able to complete IVF the number of times it required to get her.*

6) *Even though he will never know Maddie on this side of paradise, my dad knew about our journey and was able to be a part of it in the beginning.*

7) *I was able to keep my JOY for the whole journey to Maddie.*

8) *We didn't have to make any hard ethical decisions during our IVF process—God took care of that for us!*

9) *Doctors, nurses and embryologists that took time from their families and lives to receive the necessary education and took the time to help us and care for us during this whole process.*

10) *The science exists that helped us get Maddie.*

11) *I was able to be off with Maddie for 12 weeks, that is time I will never get back.*

12) *Maddie and her story are going to reach people I never could.*

13) *A husband that loves Maddie as much as I do, and will do anything for her and is a great DAD!!!*

14) *God's timing in this process, though I questioned it at times, I now see the perfection in it.*

15) *Parents that taught me to make goals and not give up on them, to fight for what I want.*

16) *My relationship with God and how much it grew during this process.*

17) *The waiting...at the time I hated it but now I know it served a purpose.*

18) *I know I will see the babies I lost someday in Heaven.*

19) *I was able to stay healthy through this journey.*

20) *God's promises...to give us the desires of our hearts and to fill us with Joy!*

21) *This holiday season that starts tomorrow and the traditions we can start with Maddie, and that this year, I have the extra stocking and the Santa picture...dreams do come true!*

22) *Maddie didn't come easy, because the journey brought me closer to God and Kevin and taught me more lessons than I could ever imagine!"*

November 22, 2018: *"Happy 1st Thanksgiving from Maddie!! Out of tradition we now kick off the Christmas season!! Christmas PJs! Kevin jokes about Maddie having so many Christmas outfits, and it's true she does have a lot. I still remember the very day I bought this sleeper...it was January 1st 2017...it was on super sale at Dillard's, and I was so sure the round of IVF we were getting ready to do would result in a baby that needed this outfit for Christmas 2017...obviously that did not happen, but almost 2 years later this outfit just so happens to be the perfect size for Maddie this Christmas season (coincidence?...I think not!! Nothing but God!). If we are faithful, he is faithful, but in his time, not ours!!! Happy Thanksgiving!!!"* **#Godandthestubblefieldskickedinfertilitysbutt #ifwearefaithfulheisfaithful**

December 3, 2018: *"Why oh why can I not live in Europe where maternity leave is 12 months?!?!?! Tomorrow I go back to work. How on Earth am I supposed to leave this girl? We have been together since January. Trying to remain thankful today...thankful I like my job* *and the people I work with, thankful I like my job and the people I work with, thankful I have had the last 12 weeks with my girl, thankful when I leave tomorrow Maddie will be in great hands and thankful that Christmas break starts in 2.5 weeks! My mom tells me going back from maternity leave was the hardest thing she had ever done up to that point in her life, while that is not true for me it is going to be a close runner up. This is how I'll be spending today... soaking up all the baby cuddles I can!! And if you see me tomorrow, don't mind the tears and maybe give me a little extra grace."*

December 4, 2018: *"Reunited and it feels so good!! In case you were wondering, I survived today! So thankful for a good job and great coworkers and my mom who took great care of Maddie!! My dad told me a long time ago...work is what we do so we can do the things we want to do! Miss that guy, but still living by his words!"*

December 12, 2018: *"3 months old today!!!! Sometimes I can't believe it and it seems like yesterday and other times it seems like I've never been without her! She is pure joy in human form! She sleeps all night and smiles all day! She has discovered her hands and loves them! She loves to talk and sing, she laughs and she gives "kisses." Oh Maddie Joy, we love you more than you will ever know! "Now all glory to God, who is able, through his mighty power at work within us, to accomplish infinitely more than we might ask or think." —Ephesians 3:20"*

December 16, 2018: *"Happy Birthday to my other half!!! We don't get all lovey-dovey on Facebook usually because we always wonder who people are trying to convince when they do that...but special days like this call for a mushy post! It's always odd to me when I really think about Kevin's and my age difference, but there is no doubt in my mind, God save him for me! He was my rock through our fight* *for Maddie, and he has always been part of my joy. He keeps me grounded. It has been a great year! Kevin is a great daddy! Maddie loves it when he holds her like a football and when he sings George Jones to her! I can't wait to see what next year brings!! Happy Birthday, Kevin Stubblefield!!"*

December 20, 2018: *"Today on the radio they were talking about the circumstances surrounding Jesus' birth…and then they said this: "God doesn't bring miracles out of perfect places, he brings miracles out of problem places." Preach it!! This little girl…my Maddie miracle did not come out of perfect places…she came out of problem places, she came out of sadness, grief, struggle, faith and perseverance. Oh what JOY fills my soul when I look at her! Whatever miracle you're wanting and praying for…know this, you don't have to have perfect circumstances, just keep fighting!!! (Sidenote: outfit courtesy of Fairy Godmother Paige Beck, who participated in the buying on faith with me and purchased this outfit many many moons ago! It never hurts to have friends who are fighting in faith with you!!)*

December 21, 2018: *"The pain that you've been feeling, can't compare to the joy that's coming. —Romans 8:18. This popped up on my memories from 2 years ago. So much truth here!! There was so much pain that Christmas and so much JOY this Christmas!!"*

December 25, 2018: *"My mantra…grief and JOY can coexist. Look at him in his pajamas…I guarantee I had to beg him to not change before opening presents. And Maddie's shirt says it all!! As great as this first Christmas was, it was very different for other reasons and it was hard, but life moves on and we must move with it. Soaking up all the joy I can with all the people I have for as long as life lets me have them. Merry Christmas!!"*

December 31, 2018: *"Oh 2018 how great you were to the Stubble-fields!! 2018 brought us Maddie Joy and there's nothing better than that! Years come and years go, they are but a blip in our whole life. Whether your year was great like ours or wasn't one of your best to-morrows we start over. In the new year remember this, fight for your JOY always and good things are coming!! Enjoy some of our moments from 2018 (sorry, not sorry for the picture overload). I'm not sure how 2019 can be better than this, but I also know our best days are before us, so bring it on!! "Take delight in the Lord, and he will give you the desires of your heart" –Psalm 37:4"*

January 12, 2019: *"This sweetheart is 4 months old today!! Today is a special day, 1 year ago today is when Maddie's embryo was im-planted in me!! Don't let anyone tell you, your circumstances can't change. The picture on the left is what Maddie looked like 1 year ago, and I don't have a picture for what my heart looked like but I can tell you it was fragile. I was placing all my hope in Jesus and believing that he had good things in store for me, but I was doubting the success of that day. We had done this so many times with so much failure. I knew that day would be our last try at IVF. 3 years' worth of effort was about to end. I remember January 12, 2018, like it was yesterday. Oddly enough it was a snow day that day too. So much has changed in 365 days…so wherever you are now you do not have to stay. Let my sweet girl and her embryo be a reminder that your cir-cumstances CAN change!! "Forget the former things; do not dwell on the past. See, I am doing a new thing!" –Isaiah 3 18-19."*

January 15, 2019: *"This cutie pie turned 4 months old on Sat-urday! She weighs 12lbs 11oz and is 24.25 inches long. She is the best baby! She loves Minnie mouse and Sophie the giraffe, she has found her hands and loves them! She can roll from belly to back, loves the Wonky Donkey book, gives kisses, loves to sing and smiles all the* *time!! I'm not sure how I lived without her, but I know this my JOY is full!! "These things I have spoken to you, that my joy may be in you, and that your joy may be full." —John 15:11"*

February 12, 2019: *"Oh my sweet, sweet Maddie girl!! 5 months old today!!! I say it every time but I seriously don't know how I lived without her. She truly is full of JOY!! She is really starting to love Kam! She can roll all directions, she loves her pineapple and Sophie the giraffe, she loves to read books and sing! She weighs almost 14 lbs. and loves all food except peas! "For his anger is but for a moment, and his favor is for a lifetime. Weeping may tarry for the night, but JOY comes with the morning." —Psalm 30:5"*

February 22, 2019: *"5 years ago today I said yes! I remember that Sonic parking lot like it was yesterday. We had no idea what marriage was. We had no idea the mountains we would climb, the valleys we would walk through, the sadness we would experience or the struggles…but we also had no idea the blessings that were coming our way! I would say yes all over again!! (Also we look like babies…so apparently marriage ages you!)"*

March 12, 2019: *"1/2 a year old!! I must quit blinking! Happy 6 months Maddie girl!! I can't believe she isn't my tiny baby anymore, but I'm loving this big girl!! I love the noises, the kisses, the playing and the smiling is my favorite!!! This girl smiles all the time!! She rolls around like a boss and would love to crawl, but just hasn't quite figured it out yet. She can sit up and put her paci in without help! Our doc appt isn't for a couple weeks so I'm not sure of her stats, but she weighs close to 15 lbs. and she is full of JOY! And I can't wait to see what the next ½ year brings! "These things I have spoken to you, that my JOY may be in you and that your JOY may be full." —John 15:11"*

April 12, 2019: *"Oh my sweet sweet girl!!! How are you closer to one year old than a newborn?!?!?! Happy 7 months Maddie girl!!!! Everything about her is perfect! She's a petite thing weighing in at 14 lbs. 10 oz and 25 in long, but I assure you she loves to eat any food you will give her! She is so so close to crawling and loves to chew on everything…today is also…another milestone for our sweet girl…2 years ago today the eff that made Maddie girl was retrieved from me… that egg would go on to spend 9 months in the freezer and another 9 months in me before it created my sweet girl and Kevin and I would face terrible heartbreak and rock bottom before we came out on the mountain top! God knew exactly what was in store for us on that day 2 years ago and I'm so glad he is in charge and not me!!!"*

April 24, 2019: *"It's National Infertility Awareness Week, and I don't really like to dwell in our infertility but rather bask in the joy of Maddie, but I wanted to acknowledge it because it will always, always be part of our story. I don't hate infertility (oh trust me there was a time when I did), I am thankful for infertility. Infertility taught me lessons I could have never learned about myself, about Kevin, about God, but most of all it taught me to find true JOY in the journey! We fought for Maddie!!!! "Every good and perfect gift is from above…" — James 1:17"*

May 12, 2019: "Oh my sweet sweet Maddie girl!! Happy 8 months sweet girl! It still blows my mind that we are knocking so close to 1! I love everything about every stage so I'm just soaking it all in. Maddie loves to eat food, "talks" all the time, can officially crawl but prefers to army crawl because it is faster, is starting to try to stand up and claps!! I don't know what I did without her!!!"

June 12, 2019: *"Oh my sweet, sweet Maddie girl!! 9 months old today!! 9 months in the freezer, 9 months in my belly and 9 months in* *our arms!! It is going so fast but I love every stage. Maddie weighs 16 lbs. and is 26.5 inches long. She can crawl anywhere she wants to go and is starting to pull up. She loves to play, loves to blow raspberries and loves to smile!!!"*

June 18, 2019: *"THIS!!! This is why I made a major life change in 2018!! When I took the job I have now, I took it for this! To be home in the summer, to spend my time with Maddie!! (No I wasn't even pregnant yet). When I took this job it was a major change, Kevin talked me into it. I was leery, I specifically remember saying to Kevin what if I am home summer after summer without a child…BUT GOD, but God knew Maddie would be coming. Sometimes you have to make the changes and make the hard choices that are best for your dream before your dream ever happens!! I am beyond grateful to be a working mom that still gets so much time with her baby and thankful for a husband that works hard so I can do this, and who is the reason I ever pursued this job!! Put feet on your dreams, prepare for what you want and find your JOY!!"*

July 12, 2019: *"This sweet, sweet girl is 10 months old today!! We are getting so close to the 1-year mark and I can't believe it. She is the best girl! She loves to play, she is furniture walking, she is climbing, she loves to read and gives awesome kisses! I'm enjoying every second of my summer with her!!"*

August 12, 2019: *"How oh how are you 11 months old today sweet Maddie?!?! I can't believe the next time I make a post like this she will be a WHOLE year old. She loves to smile, loves to wave at everyone, and loves to read (that makes this mama's heart so happy). She gives her baby dolls hugs and still gives awesome kisses. She is cruising everywhere but just isn't quite ready to let go. I love her more than I can* *explain!! I'm so blessed I got to spend the last 12 weeks at home with her! I am going to miss her like crazy com Friday!"*

September 11, 2019: *"Heaven blew every trumpet and played every horn on the wonderful, marvelous night you were born." "Prepare for post overload over the next few days as we spend the rest of this week and weekend celebrating our girl! Tonight I put to bed a baby and tomorrow she wakes up a 1-year-old! Oh the night she was born, I will always treasure that memory, a room full of people took a collective deep breath when Maddie breathed her first. We had a healthy, perfect baby! Our family grew instead of shrank! She is my miracle baby in every sense of the word, her story will reach people I never could have and I believe she will do great things! I can't imagine what life would be like if I would have quit fighting for her! Happy birthday my sweet Maddie Joy!!!"*

THE FIRST YEAR IS FULL OF FIRSTS, JOY AND LESSONS

Maddie's first year of life taught me so much—probably more than I will ever teach her. I know that every person that ever has a baby thinks that baby is perfect for them (and they probably are)—but Maddie was perfect for Kevin and I's circumstances. Maddie was the easiest baby—and I think God knew there were things Kevin and I needed in a baby and he was sure to provide them with Maddie. She was a sleeper from day one—she never had colic, she seriously rarely cried—she was probably as low maintenance as a newborn could be.

My life will always be defined as before Maddie and after Maddie. She will always be my tangible reminder that God can do infinitely more than we might think or understand. Struggles came to us after Maddie—financially, in our marriage, in Kevin's health—in a variety of ways—but it was so much easier for me to pray and believe God for those things when I looked at Maddie and remembered the days I thought I may never have her.

A few months after Maddie was born—due to some legal problems for the agency, we ended up getting almost a full refund on the money we paid to our adoption agency—money that when we paid we were warned would not ever be refunded for ANY reason. I truly feel like God wanted to know if we were truly willing to take that step of faith—to see if we really wanted it that bad—and when we did he provided in more ways than one.

I don't exactly know when it was—maybe the day we came home from the hospital (HAHA—not that soon), or maybe when Maddie was 6 months or so I started thinking about never having another baby—I knew from the day they put Maddie's embryo in me that it was my last shot at having a baby, that I would never do it again and I truly tried to soak up every ounce and second of my pregnancy—but my woman and mama heart couldn't help but let my mind wander there. The problems though are too numerous to count—for instance even if we could have afforded another IVF cycle—what if they retrieved 5 or 6 eggs from me and they all worked—while I would have loved to have another baby—I could NOT have 5 babies. When I thought truthfully about the problems I could have had with Maddie—what if I would have needed bed rest or a C section—those things would have been very, very difficult for Kevin and I's circumstances. Having another baby was just not in the cards for me—which I'm not going to lie is something I still struggle with frequently, but that's just it…infertility never stops and never will, grief never stops… and never will, sadness never stops…and never will, tragedy never stops…and never will…you see where I'm going here…but we must always, always CHOOSE JOY!!

I am one of the blessed ones—I won my fight for infertility and I learned to continuously win my fight for JOY—it is easier as I hold Maddie Joy in my arms every day and she truly is a tangible form of answered prayers—promises fulfilled and JOY in human form!! I hope that her story reaches others who are struggling… and I hope that it fulfills my promise, I promised long ago to GOD that I would share my story—that I would make sure people knew what he DID for ME!! So here's your reminder that God is no respecter of persons and what he did for me, he can do for you—and maybe you don't need a Maddie Joy—maybe you need, financial security or peace in your marriage or whatever it is you need…learn to find JOY while you fight for it!!

"And we know that in all things God works for the good of those who love him, who have been called according to his purpose."
—Romans 8:28

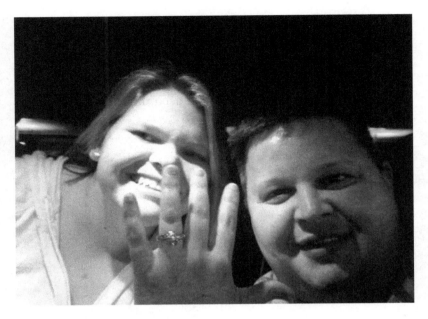

1. The night Kevin asked me to marry him in the Sonic parking lot

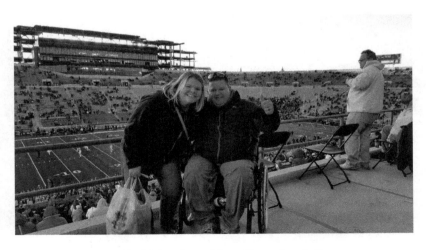

2. Kevin and Mariah at a Notre Dame Football game

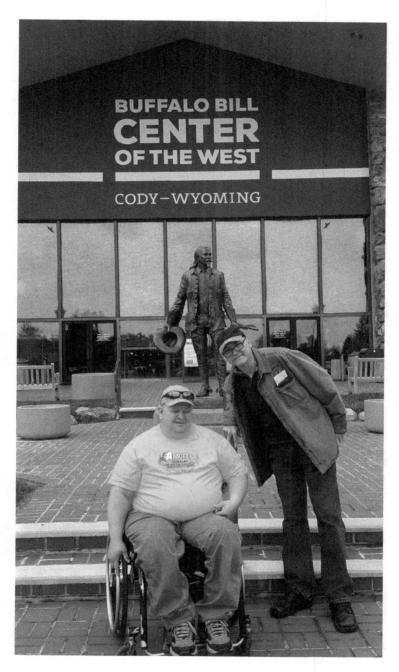

3. Kevin and my dad on our family vacation- taken 2 days before he died

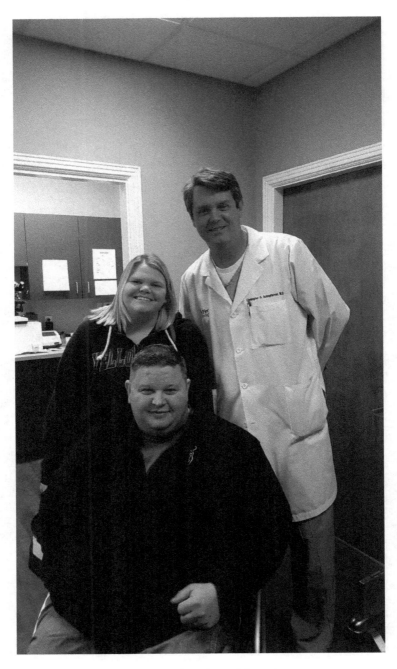

4. Kevin, Mariah and Dr. Schrepferman

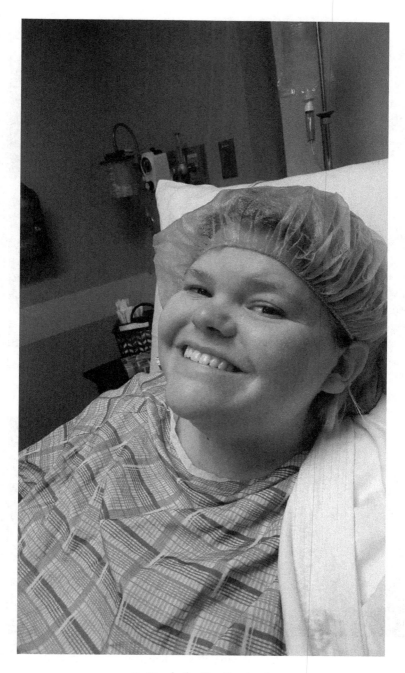

5. Ready for Egg Retrieval

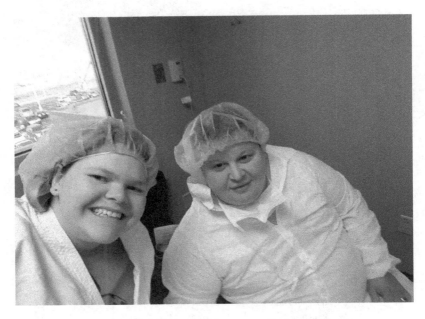

6. Ready for Implantation- Kevin really loved the suit!

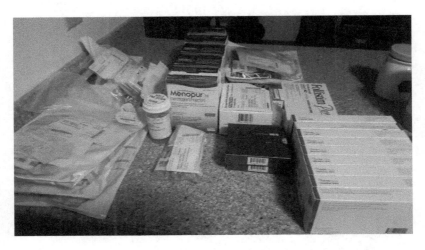

7. "Baby in a Box"- Medicine

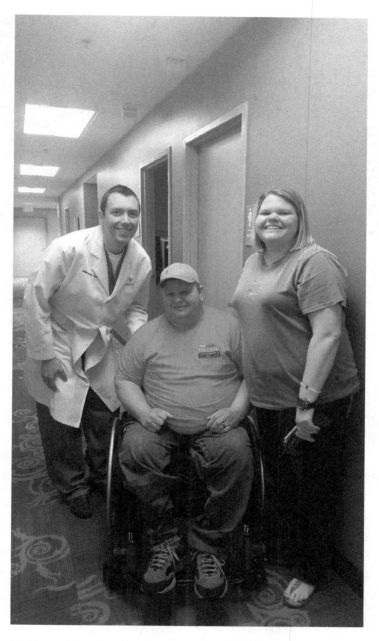

8. Kevin, Mariah and Dr. Griffin the day we were released from his care for our boy- who knew we would be back in less than 2 weeks under much different circumstances

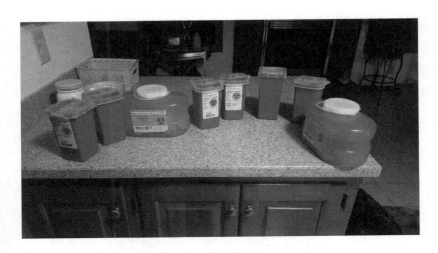

9. Needles!!

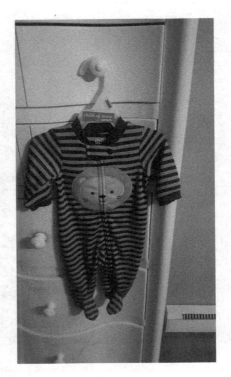

10. The lion sleeper hung in this spot for YEARS!

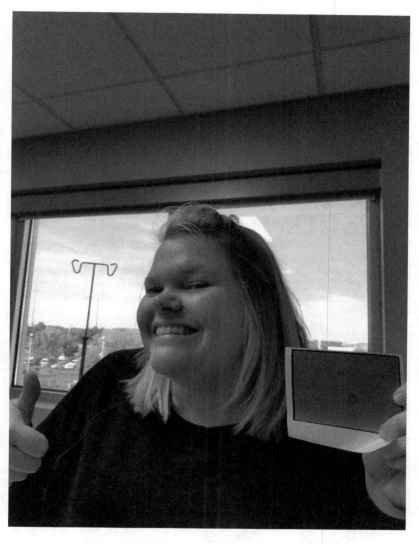

11. Post transfer with a baby I would never hold

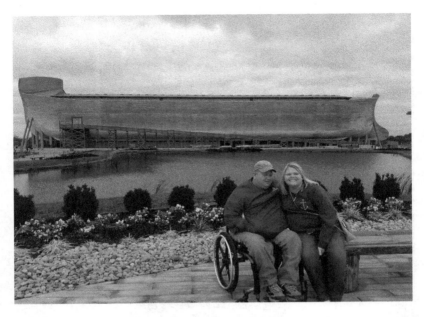

12. Kevin and Mariah on vacation to The Ark

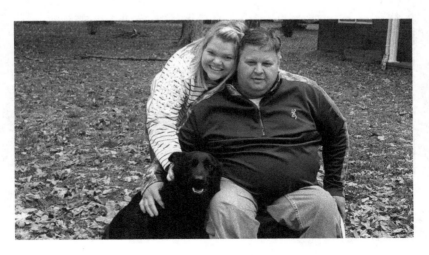

13. Our adoption profile picture

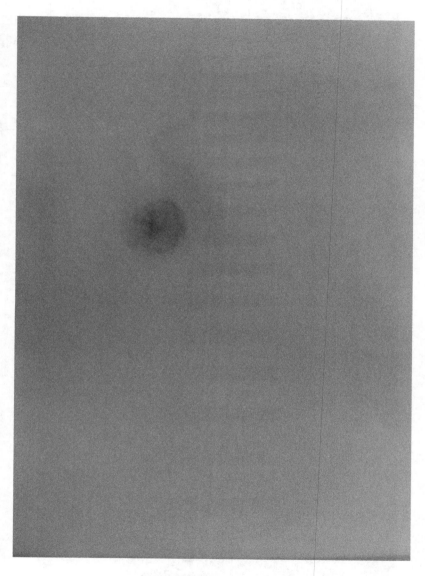

14. Maddie's first baby picture!

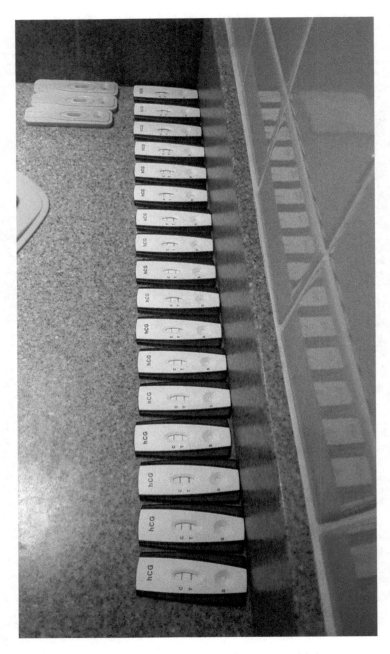

15. Pee on a stick Marathon- These are Maddie's!

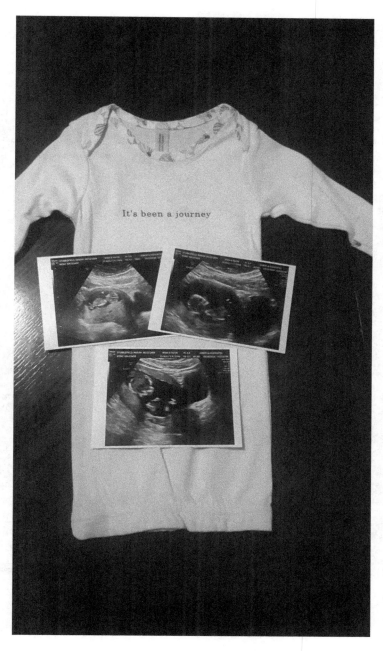

16. Maddie's Pregnancy announcement- This gown was at least 2 years old by the time we used it here

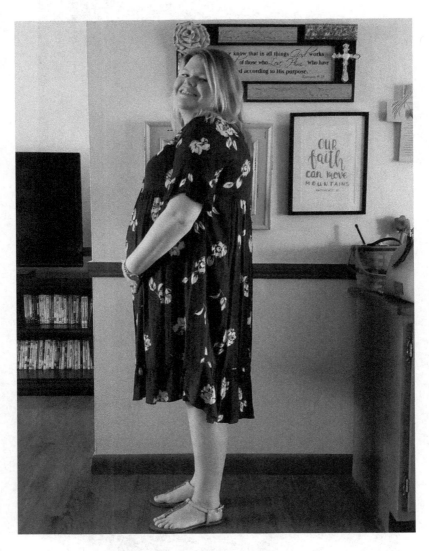

17. 1st Bump picture!

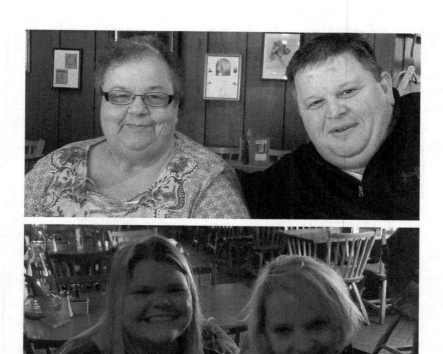

18. Each of us with our moms the day we found out Maddie was a Girl!

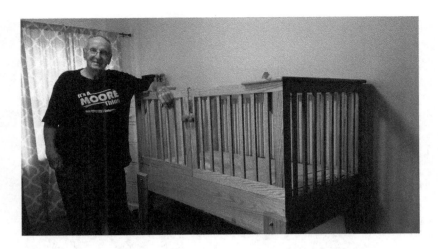

19. My Grandpa standing next to the crib he built us both with wood and screws but also prayers

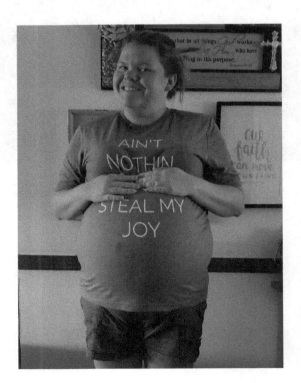

20. Me sporting my favorite shirt and a bump!

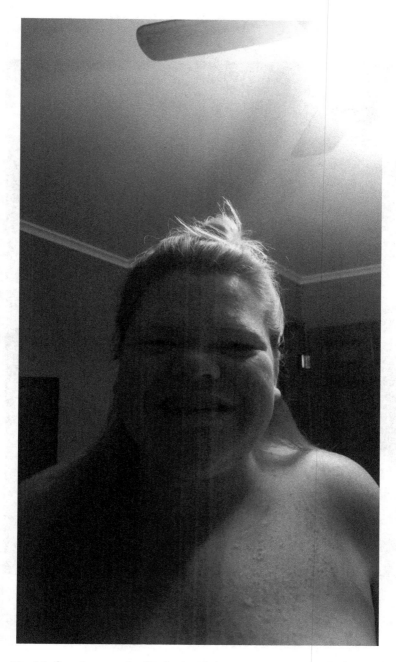

21. My face the morning Kevin decided it was time to go to the hospital

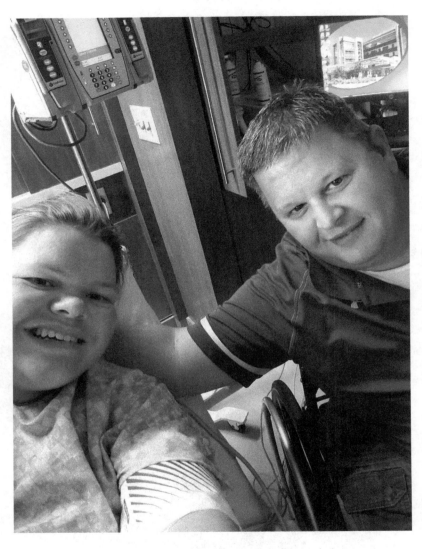

22. Kevin and Mariah getting ready to have a baby!

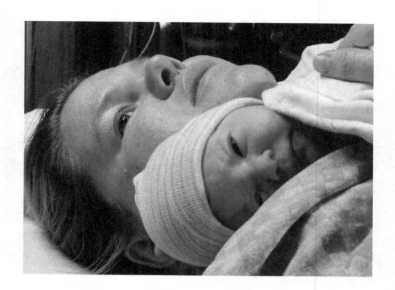

23. The first time I held Maddie

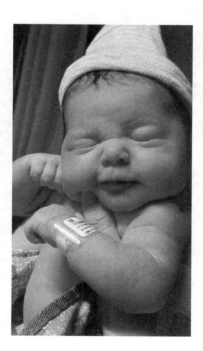

24. Sweet Maddie girl is perfect!

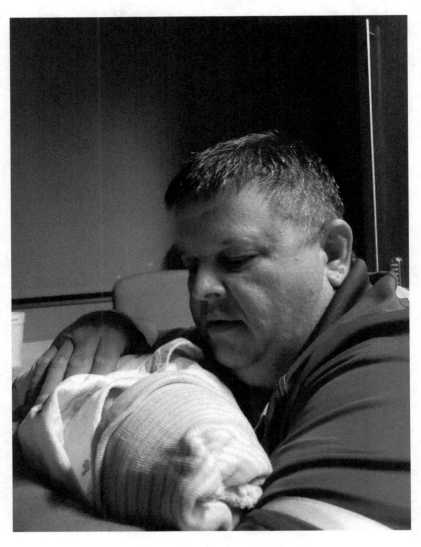

25. The first time Kevin held Maddie

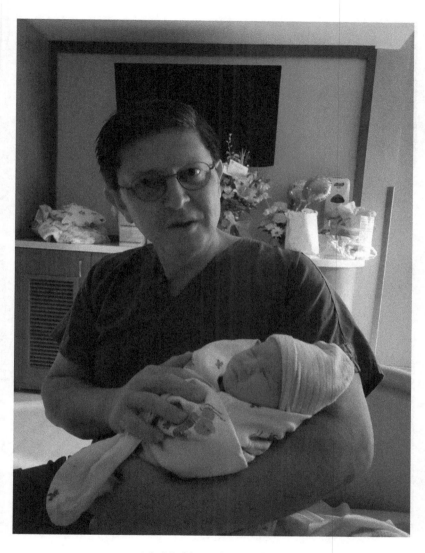

26. Maddie and Dr. Asbery

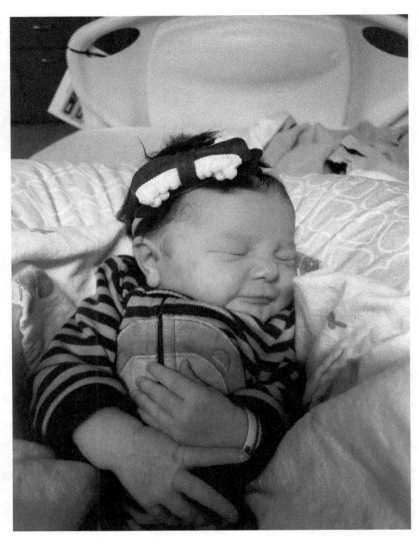

27. The lion sleeper is finally getting worn!

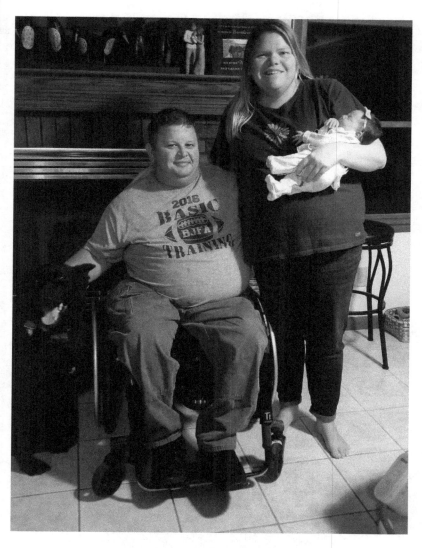

28. Our first family photo

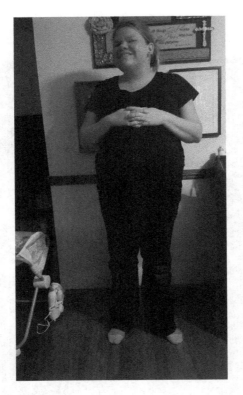

29. The last bump picture- taken the night before we went to the hospital

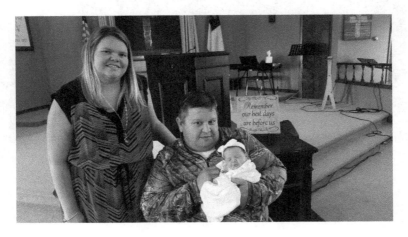

30. Maddie's baby dedication

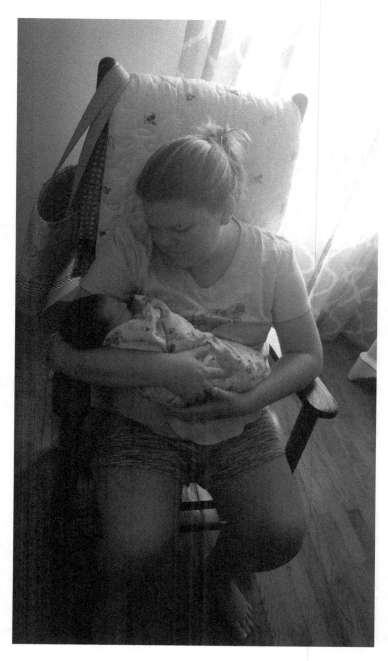

31. Me and Maddie our first full day at home

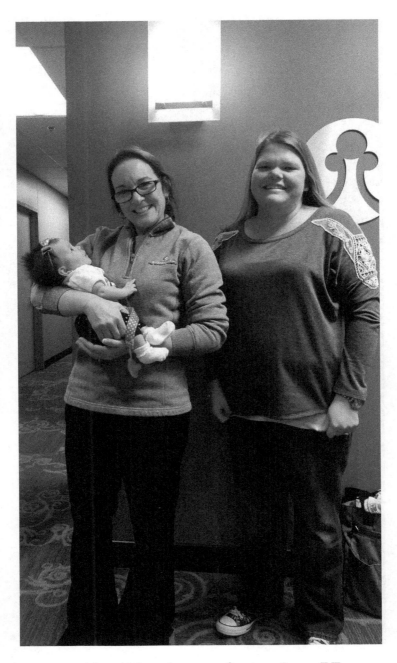

32. Me and Missy- she was my favorite at Boston IVF

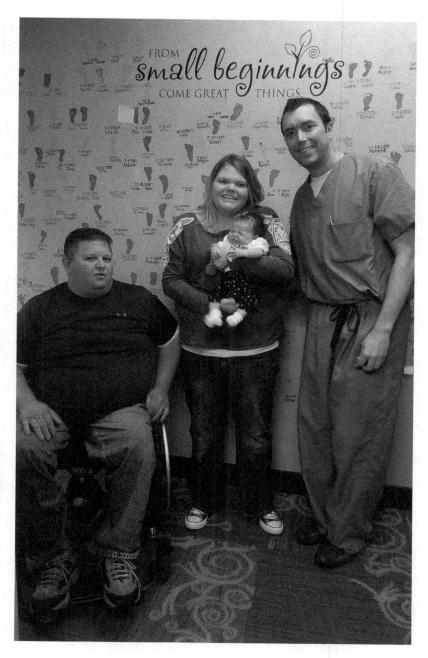

33. Us and Dr. Griffin in front of the footprint wall "The Victory Lap"

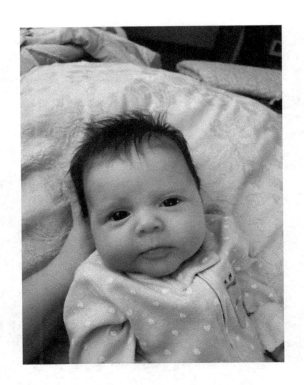

34. Sweet Maddie girl

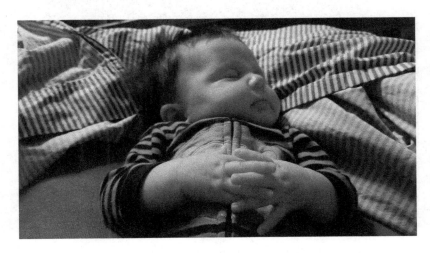

35. Maddie!

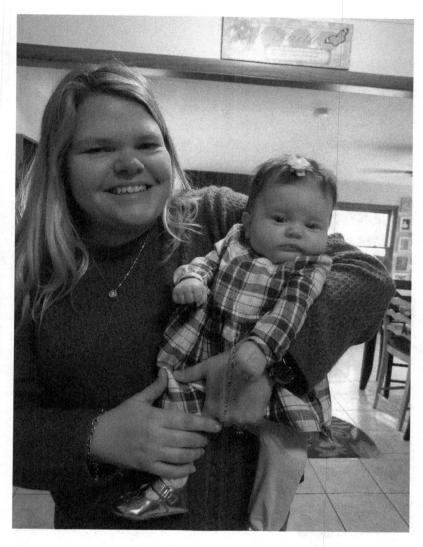

36. Maddie and Mariah!

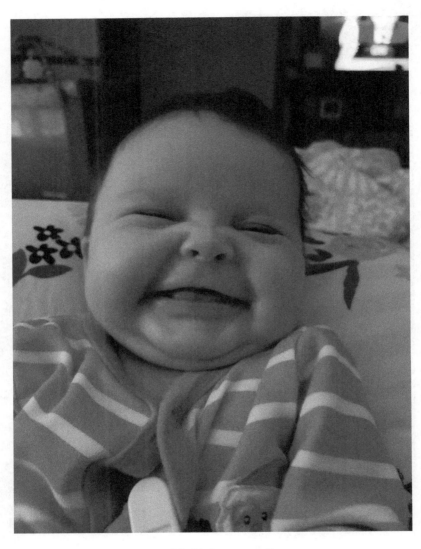

37. Maddie's sweet smile

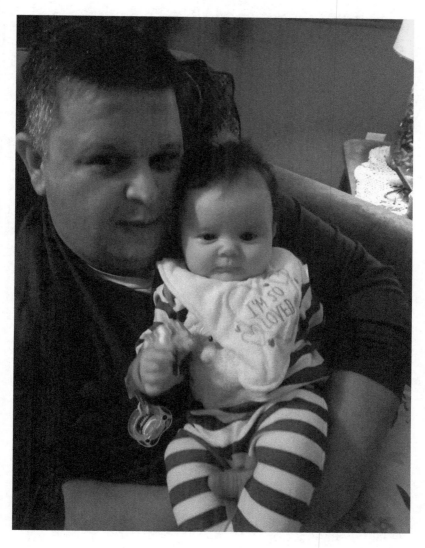

38. Kevin and Maddie

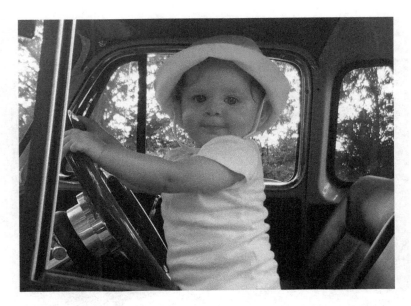

39. Maddie girl

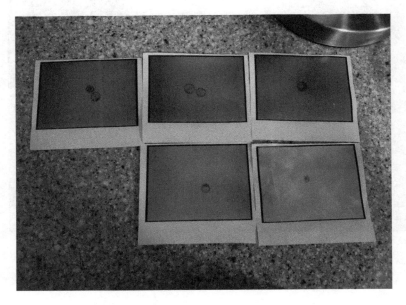

40. 7 of our 11 babies- I will always love every one of them-
They all taught me something

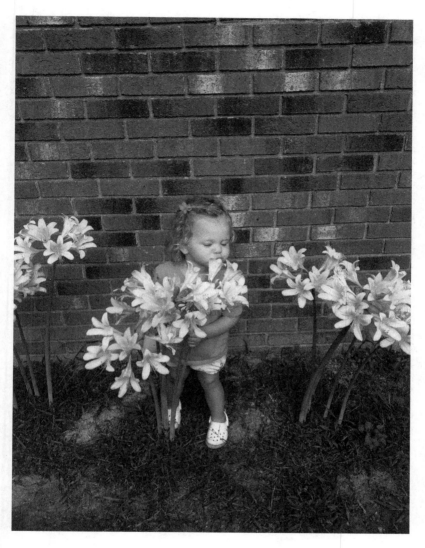

41. Maddie with our Magic Lilies- they always remind
me that circumstances can quickly change.

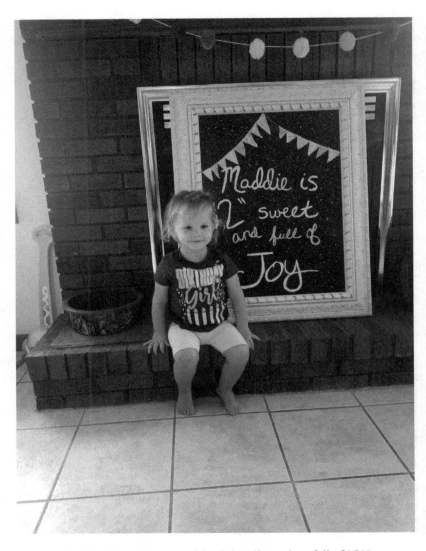

42. Maddie on her second birthday! She truly is full of JOY!